MCQs for
Anesthesiology Postgraduates
for DM Entrance Examinees

MCQs for Anesthesiology Postgraduates
for DM Entrance Examinees

Editors

Atul Prabhakar Kulkarni
MD (Anesthesiology) FISCCM PGDHHM FICCM
Professor and Head
Division of Critical Care Medicine
Department of Anesthesiology, Critical Care and Pain
Tata Memorial Hospital
Homi Bhabha National Institute
Mumbai, Maharashtra, India

Madhavi Desai
DA DNB (Anesthesiology)
Associate Professor
Department of Anesthesiology, Critical Care and Pain
Tata Memorial Hospital
Homi Bhabha National Institute
Mumbai, Maharashtra, India

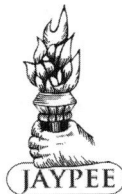

JAYPEE BROTHERS MEDICAL PUBLISHERS
The Health Sciences Publisher
New Delhi | London

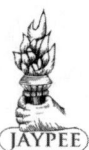
Jaypee Brothers Medical Publishers (P) Ltd

Headquarters
Jaypee Brothers Medical Publishers (P) Ltd
EMCA House, 23/23-B
Ansari Road, Daryaganj
New Delhi 110 002, India
Landline: +91-11-23272143, +91-11-23272703
+91-11-23282021, +91-11-23245672
Email: jaypee@jaypeebrothers.com

Corporate Office
Jaypee Brothers Medical Publishers (P) Ltd
4838/24, Ansari Road, Daryaganj
New Delhi 110 002, India
Phone: +91-11-43574357
Fax: +91-11-43574314
Email: jaypee@jaypeebrothers.com

Overseas Office
JP Medical Ltd
83 Victoria Street, London
SW1H 0HW (UK)
Phone: +44 20 3170 8910
Fax: +44 (0)20 3008 6180
Email: info@jpmedpub.com

Website: www.jaypeebrothers.com
Website: www.jaypeedigital.com

© 2023, Jaypee Brothers Medical Publishers

The views and opinions expressed in this book are solely those of the original contributor(s)/author(s) and do not necessarily represent those of editor(s) or publisher of the book.

All rights reserved. No part of this publication may be reproduced, stored or transmitted in any form or by any means, electronic, mechanical, photocopying, recording or otherwise, without the prior permission in writing of the publishers.

All brand names and product names used in this book are trade names, service marks, trademarks or registered trademarks of their respective owners. The publisher is not associated with any product or vendor mentioned in this book.

Medical knowledge and practice change constantly. This book is designed to provide accurate, authoritative information about the subject matter in question. However, readers are advised to check the most current information available on procedures included and check information from the manufacturer of each product to be administered, to verify the recommended dose, formula, method and duration of administration, adverse effects and contraindications. It is the responsibility of the practitioner to take all appropriate safety precautions. Neither the publisher nor the author(s)/editor(s) assume any liability for any injury and/or damage to persons or property arising from or related to use of material in this book.

This book is sold on the understanding that the publisher is not engaged in providing professional medical services. If such advice or services are required, the services of a competent medical professional should be sought.

Every effort has been made where necessary to contact holders of copyright to obtain permission to reproduce copyright material. If any have been inadvertently overlooked, the publisher will be pleased to make the necessary arrangements at the first opportunity.

Inquiries for bulk sales may be solicited at: jaypee@jaypeebrothers.com

MCQs for Anesthesiology Postgraduates for DM Entrance Examinees

First Edition: **2023**

ISBN: 978-93-5465-955-3

Printed at: Rajkamal Electric Press, Kundli, Haryana.

Dedicated to

*The warriors who study the most blessed art of anesthesia,
but remain anonymous while ensuring the patient's wellbeing.*

Contributors

Amol Kothekar MD IDCCM
Professor Intensive Care Medicine
Department of Anesthesia, Critical Care and Pain
Tata Memorial Hospital
Homi Bhabha National Institute
Mumbai, Maharashtra, India

Anjali Ashok Pingle MBBS DA DNB FRCA
Consultant
Department of Anesthesiology
PD Hinduja Hospital and Medical Research Centre
Mumbai, Maharashtra, India

Anjana Sagar Wajekar
DNB Fellowship in Neuroanaesthesiology FAIMER Fellow
Associate Professor (Anesthesiology)
Department of Anesthesiology, Critical Care and Pain
Tata Memorial Hospital
Homi Bhabha National Institute
Mumbai, Maharashtra, India

Aparna Sanjay Chatterjee MD FCARCSI (Dublin)
Professor
Department of Anesthesiology, Critical Care and Pain
Tata Memorial Hospital
Homi Bhabha National Institute
Mumbai, Maharashtra, India

Atul Prabhakar Kulkarni
MD (Anesthesiology) FISCCM PGDHHM FICCM
Professor and Head
Division of Critical Care Medicine
Department of Anesthesiology, Critical Care and Pain
Tata Memorial Hospital
Homi Bhabha National Institute
Mumbai, Maharashtra, India
Editor-in-Chief, Indian Journal of Critical Care Medicine
President Asia Pacific Association of Critical Care Medicine
Past President, Indian Society of Critical Care Medicine
Past Chancellor, Indian College of Critical Care Medicine
Past President, Association of SAARC Critical Care Societies

Bhoomika Parimal Thakore DNB PDF (Neuroanaesthesia)
Consultant
Department of Anesthesiology
PD Hinduja Hospital and Medical Research Centre
Mumbai, Maharashtra, India

Deepshikha Palit MBBS MD MRCA
ST5 Anaesthetics
Cambridge University Hospitals, UK

Ketan K Kataria MBBS MD DNB DM
Assistant Professor
Department of Anesthesiology, Critical Care and Pain
Tata Memorial Hospital
Homi Bhabha National Institute
Mumbai, Maharashtra, India

Lalita Gouri Mitra DA MD DMB MNAMS
Associate Professor
Department of Anesthesia and Critical Care
Institute of Liver and Biliary Sciences
New Delhi, India

Madhavi Desai DA DNB (Anesthesiology)
Associate Professor
Department of Anesthesiology, Critical Care and Pain
Tata Memorial Hospital
Homi Bhabha National Institute
Mumbai, Maharashtra, India

Madhavi Shetmahajan MD (Anaesthesiology) FRCA
Professor (Thoracic Anesthesia)
Department of Anesthesiology, Critical Care and Pain
Tata Memorial Centre
Homi Bhabha National Institute
Mumbai, Maharashtra, India

Mihika Jigeeshu Divatia MBBS MD (Anaesthesiology)
Senior Resident
Department of Anesthesiology, Critical Care and Pain
Tata Memorial Hospital
Homi Bhabha National Institute
Mumbai, Maharashtra, India

Mahima Gupta MBBS MD DM (Onco-anaesthesia)
Assistant Professor
Department of Anaesthesiology, Pain and Critical Care
Hamdard Institute of Medical Sciences and Research
(HIMSR) and HAHC
New Delhi, India

Nandini Malay Dave MD DNB (Anesthesia) MNAMS
Senior Consultant and Head
Department of Pediatric Anesthesia
SRCC NH Children's Hospital
Mumbai, Maharashtra, India

Nirmalyo Lodh
MBBS MD MRCP (UK) DM (Critical Care Medicine) EDIC EDAIC
Severe Respiratory Failure and ECMO Fellow
Intensive Care Medicine
Guy's and St Thomas NHS Foundation Trust, London UK

Nupur Karan MD (Anaesthesiology) DM (Neuroanaesthesiology)
Assistant Professor
Department of Anesthesiology
Kalinga Institute of Medical Sciences
Bhubaneswar, Odisha, India

Riddhi Joshi MD (Anaesthesiology)
Trainee of Australia and New Zealand College of Anaesthetists
and Registrar in Anaesthesia
Dubbo Base Hospital
New South Wales, Australia

Sheetal Vidyadhar Gaikwad
MD (Anesthesia) Fellowship in Regional Anaesthesia and Airway, Germany
Associate Professor
Department of Anesthesiology, Critical Care and Pain
Tata Memorial Hospital
Mumbai, Maharashtra, India

Shruti Gairola
MD (Anesthesia) KGMU, Lucknow DM (Onco-anaesthesia) AIIMS, New Delhi
Assistant Professor
Department of Anesthesiology, Critical Care and Pain
Tata Memorial Hospital
Homi Bhabha National Institute
Mumbai, Maharashtra, India

Sneha Toal MD DNB (Anaesthesiology)
Postgraduate Resident Medical Officer
BARC Hospital
Mumbai, Maharashtra, India

Sukhada Dhananjay Savarkar MBBS MD
Associate Professor
Department of Anesthesiology,
Critical Care and Pain
Tata Memorial Hospital
Homi Bhabha National Institute
Mumbai, Maharashtra, India

Sumitra Ganesh Bakshi MD DNB (Anesthesia)
Professor (Anesthesia, Critical Care and Pain)
Department of Anesthesiology,
Critical Care and Pain
Tata Memorial Hospital
Homi Bhabha National Institute
Mumbai, Maharashtra, India

Swati Rajen Daftary MBBS DA MD
Senior Consultant
Department of Anesthesia and Pain Management
Sir HN Reliance Foundation Hospital
Mumbai, Maharashtra, India

Vandana Saluja
MBBS MD (Anesthesia) PDCC Liver Transplant Anesthesia
Additional Professor and Senior Consultant
Department of Anesthesia and Critical Care
Amrita Institute of Medical Sciences
Faridabad, Haryana, India

Preface

Do you know what it means to relieve man of his pain and suffering? Anesthesia is the most humane of all of man's accomplishments, and what a merciful accomplishment it was. For this great discovery, we are indebted to Dr WTG Morton.

—**Joseph Lewis in the book 'An Atheist Manifesto'**

It gives us great pleasure to bring to you the first edition of *MCQs for Anesthesiology Postgraduates for DM Entrance Examinees*. Advancement in surgical techniques and super-specialization in various surgical branches, it was a given that a similar trend will emerge in the vast discipline of Anesthesia. Today we have anesthesia super-specialization in various fields such as Solid Organ Transplant Anesthesia, Neuro-Anesthesia, Pediatric Anesthesia, etc., all these "Superspecialists" resulting in many advances and importantly improvement in patient outcomes. Nowadays, you cannot pursue any discipline without clearing the essential hurdle of entrance examinations. When you prepare for this trial by fire, you need help to train the mind in critical and quick thinking, which hopefully this book will help in.

This book therefore, contains multiple choice questions (MCQs) dealing with many disciplines essential for the anesthesia postgraduates who is preparing for leaping this hurdle before entering the rarified environment of superspecialty practice. As always the reader is the best judge of the utility of the book. All answers to the MCQs are supported by references from either a standard textbook or an article published in a PubMed Indexed Journal. We hope you get back to us with suggestions and criticisms, so that we can improve the next edition! We wish all postgraduates a happy reading and success in their examination!

Atul Prabhakar Kulkarni
Madhavi Desai

Acknowledgments

We wish to acknowledge the help of all the authors for their valuable time, and their keenness in setting the questions, writing the explanations for the chosen answers, for the readers to improve their understanding. They made it possible for us to bring out this book. The students in the discipline of anesthesia, who inspire us to teach, the readers, deserve our thanks.

We are especially thankful to Shri Jitendar P Vij (Group Chairman), Mr Ankit Vij (Managing Director), Mr MS Mani (Group President), Ms Chetna Malhotra (Senior Director–Professional Publishing, Marketing and Business Development), and Ms Saima Rashid (Manager Publishing) of M/s Jaypee Brothers Medical Publishers (P) Ltd, New Delhi, India, for giving a go-ahead at the very beginning and helping us in every way possible to bring out this book. Last but not least, our prayers and thanks to the Almighty for blessing us in this task.

Contents

Multiple Choice Questions and Answers with Explanation

Questions 1

Answers 54

Multiple Choice Questions and Answers with Explanation

QUESTIONS

1. The global cerebral blood flow (CBF) in adults is:
   a. 25 mL/100 g/min
   b. 50 mL/100 g/min
   c. 100 mL/100 g/min
   d. 150 mL/100 g/min

2. What will be the cerebral perfusion pressure (CPP) (mm Hg) of a patient with mean arterial pressure (MAP) of 80 mm Hg, intracranial pressure (ICP) of 10 mm Hg and central venous pressure (CVP) of 15 mm Hg?
   a. 70
   b. 65
   c. 55
   d. 57

3. Which intravenous anesthetic agent does not decrease CBF?
   a. Etomidate
   b. Propofol
   c. Ketamine
   d. Thiopental

4. Which of the following agents has the least effect on somatosensory-evoked potentials (SSEPs)?
   a. Rocuronium
   b. Propofol
   c. Fentanyl
   d. Sevoflurane

5. The electrophysiological monitor most resistant to anesthetic agents is:
   a. Somatosensory-evoked potentials
   b. Motor-evoked potentials
   c. Electroencephalography
   d. Brainstem auditory-evoked potentials (BAEP)

6. What is *true* regarding the acute management of a subarachnoid hemorrhage (SAH)?
   a. The peak incidence of vasospasm occurs at day 4
   b. Intravenous magnesium reduces the incidence of vasospasm
   c. Hypervolemia, hypertension and hemodilution therapy reduces the incidence of vasospasm
   d. Mean arterial pressure (MAP) targets should be set to >90 mm Hg following clipping of the aneurysm

7. Which of the following tests helps confirm the diagnosis of brainstem death?
   a. Sluggishly reacting pupils
   b. Absent visual evoked responses alone
   c. Absent cough reflex response to bronchial stimulation by a suction catheter placed down the trachea to the carina
   d. Absent motor response to a sternal rub

8. Which of the following is considered as a risk factor for aneurysmal SAH?
   a. Male gender
   b. Ehlers-Danlos syndrome
   c. Pregnancy
   d. Hypotension

9. Which of the following statements is *incorrect* in context to a trauma patient with a high cervical spine injury?
   a. There is progressive bradycardia and hypotension due to the developing spinal shock
   b. In the hypotensive patient, hemorrhage should be sought and excluded as a matter of priority
   c. A MAP of 90 mm Hg is advised to optimize cord perfusion
   d. Abdominal breathing is a sign of impending respiratory deterioration

10. What is *true* regarding ICP monitoring?
    a. Lundberg A waves are normal
    b. P1 represents the dicrotic notch correlating with the closure of the aortic valve
    c. P2 corresponds to transmission of the venous pressure from the choroid plexus
    d. When the amplitude of P2 exceeds P1 this is suggestive of reduced brain compliance

11. Which statement is *true* regarding vascular access during cardiopulmonary resuscitation (CPR)?
    a. Peripherally injected drugs should be flushed with at least 20 mL of fluid followed by arm raise
    b. Drug doses should be doubled if delivered via the intraosseous route
    c. Tracheal drug administration is recommended route if intravenous route not possible
    d. Flow rates are higher when intraosseous access is secured in the tibia than the humerus

12. Which of the following cannot be used to lower the ICP in a patient undergoing craniotomy for subdural hematoma?
    a. Mannitol
    b. Hyperventilation
    c. Steroids
    d. Furosemide

13. After providing a shock with an automated external defibrillator (AED) you should:
    a. Start CPR, beginning with chest compressions
    b. Check pulse
    c. Give a rescue breath
    d. Let the AED reanalyze the rhythm

14. During CPR with no advanced airway in place the compression-to-ventilation ratio is:
    a. 5:1
    b. 30:2
    c. 10:1
    d. 20:2

15. The basic life support (BLS) assessment focuses on:
    a. Early CPR and early defibrillation
    b. Early use of advanced airways and drugs
    c. Rapid access to emergency services
    d. Proper rhythm interpretation

16. Which of the following statement would not be ideal for effective resuscitation team dynamics?
    a. Team leaders and team members should have clear, closed-loop communication
    b. Team members inform the team leader when a task begins or ends
    c. Team members do not question team leaders orders even if doubt exists
    d. Team leaders define all roles of team members in the clinical setting

17. Which of the following is performed before the BLS assessment?
    a. Make sure the scene is safe
    b. Activate EMS and get an AED if available
    c. Tap the victim's shoulder and say "Are you alright?"
    d. Call for help

18. Which of the following is the *correct* sequence of steps for BLS CPR?
    a. Chest compressions, airway, breathing
    b. Airway, breathing, circulation
    c. Circulation, airway, breathing
    d. Access care early, begin CPR, check pulse

19. When providing BLS/ACLS to a known or suspected cervical spine trauma which of the following is *incorrect* when attempting to open the airway?
    a. Open the airway using the jaw thrust without head extension
    b. Use a head tilt-chin lift maneuver if the jaw thrust is not effective
    c. Use manual restriction to stabilize the head
    d. Use an immobilization device to stabilize the head

20. During the (C) circulation portion of the Primary Assessment, the following actions are carried out:
    a. Look, listen, and feel
    b. Obtain IV access, attach ECG leads, monitor rhythm, given medications to manage rhythm, give IV/IO fluids if needed
    c. Obtain IV access, give supplemental oxygen, secure the advanced airway, give IV/IO fluids if needed
    d. Check a pulse, monitor heart rhythm, begin CPR if indicated

21. In the Primary Assessment of the systematic approach to ACLS, the D stands for:
    a. Defibrillation
    b. Definitive care
    c. Differential diagnosis
    d. Disability

22. Which drugs are involved in the bradycardia algorithm as per the recent CPR guidelines?
    a. Atropine, epinephrine, dopamine
    b. Atropine, norepinephrine, dopamine
    c. Atropine, lidocaine, adenosine
    d. Atropine, epinephrine, lidocaine

23. The *correct* dose of dopamine recommended in the bradycardia algorithm as per the recent CPR guidelines is:
    a. 5–20 mcg/kg/min infusion
    b. 2–8 mcg/kg/min infusion
    c. 5–10 mcg/kg/min infusion
    d. 1–5 mcg/kg/min infusion

24. The *correct* dose of atropine given in the bradycardia algorithm is:
    a. 1 mg atropine, may repeat up to a total dose of 3 mg
    b. 0.5 mg atropine, may repeat up to a total dose of 2 mg
    c. 0.5 mg atropine, may repeat up to a total dose of 3 mg
    d. 1 mg atropine, may repeat up to a total dose of 4 mg

25. Which of the following are treated with synchronized shocks?
    a. Unstable atrial fibrillation
    b. Sinus tachycardia
    c. VT without a pulse
    d. VF

26. Which of these is NOT a recommended pharmacological treatment for a stable patient with a wide complex ventricular tachycardia (monomorphic)?
    a. Epinephrine
    b. Sotalol
    c. Amiodarone
    d. Procainamide

27. Where should you palpate for a pulse on an unconscious infant during CPR?
    a. Radial pulse
    b. Brachial pulse
    c. Femoral pulse
    d. Carotid pulse

28. A 36-year-old woman has palpitations, lightheadedness, and a stable tachycardia. The monitor shows a regular narrow-complex QRS at a rate of 180/min. Vagal maneuvers have not been effective in terminating the rhythm. An IV has been established. What drug should be administered IV?
    a. Epinephrine 2–10 µg/kg per minute
    b. Atropine 0.5 mg
    c. Lidocaine 1 mg/kg
    d. Adenosine 6 mg

29. A patient is in cardiac arrest. High-quality chest compression are being given. The patient is intubated and an IV has been established. The rhythm is asystole. The first drug/dose to be administered is:
    a. Epinephrine 3 mg via ETT
    b. Dopamine 2–20 µg/kg per minute IV
    c. Atropine 1 mg IV
    d. Epinephrine 1 mg IV

30. A patient is in pulseless VT. Two shocks and one dose of epinephrine have been given. The next drug/dose to anticipate to administer is:
    a. Vasopressin 40 U
    b. Lidocaine 0.5 mg/kg
    c. Epinephrine 3 mg
    d. Amiodarone 300 mg

31. Which of the following will not be seen in a patient with air embolism?
    a. Hypertension
    b. Heart murmur
    c. Arrhythmia
    d. Decreased EtCO$_2$

32. Most sensitive method to detect air embolism is:
    a. Transesophageal echocardiogram (TEE)
    b. Decreased end-tidal carbon dioxide
    c. Increased end-tidal nitrogen
    d. Mill wheel murmur

33. Where should the transducer of the arterial line be zeroed in a patient undergoing craniotomy?
    a. Level of hypothalamus
    b. Level of heart
    c. Level of external auditory meatus
    d. Level of atmosphere

34. What is *true* regarding cerebrospinal fluid (CSF)?
    a. It is formed in the third ventricle
    b. It is absorbed in arachnoid granulations present in fourth ventricle
    c. Total volume of CSF is about 150 mL
    d. Major mechanism of formation is by passive diffusion of ions

35. Which of the following will not be seen in a patient with Acromegaly?
    a. Hypotension
    b. Obstructive sleep apnea
    c. Difficult airway
    d. Hyperglycemia

36. Which of the following statements regarding Glasgow Coma Scale (GCS) is *true*?
    a. The minimum score is 0
    b. A GCS of 10 means the patient is in coma
    c. Eye opening to command/speech is scored as 2
    d. A GCS of 6 means the patient is in coma

37. When does primary brain injury occur?
    a. At the moment of impact
    b. In the first hour after injury
    c. In the first 4 h after injury
    d. In the first 24 h after injury

38. Cerebral autoregulation maintains normal CBF in what range of mean arterial blood pressures?
    a. 50–150 mm Hg
    b. 50–100 mm Hg
    c. 25–50 mm Hg
    d. 80–200 mm Hg

39. Patients with severe head injury often develop a low blood sodium level (hyponatremia). Which of the following is the cause?
    a. The syndrome of inappropriate secretion of antidiuretic hormone (SIADH)
    b. Uncontrolled diabetes insipidus
    c. Uncontrolled diabetes mellitus
    d. Excess production of cortisol

40. In what percentage of patients with head injury do late seizures (i.e. >1 week after head injury) occur?
    a. 20%
    b. 5%
    c. 50%
    d. 90 %

41. Which of the following statements regarding compartment syndrome is *true*?
    a. It is detected by a loss of distal pulses and sensation
    b. It produces pain out of all proportion to the injury
    c. It is more common in open fractures than closed ones
    d. It only occurs close to a fracture

42. Which of the following compensatory mechanism maintains normal ICP in the face of an increasing intracranial mass lesion in adults?
    a. Reduction in venous blood volume
    b. Increase in skull volume
    c. Sunsetting eyes
    d. Increase in CSF production

43. **What is the safest and most reliable way to clear the cervical spine in an unconscious patient?**
    a. Cervical spine series of plain X-rays
    b. Flexion and extension views
    c. Magnetic resonance imaging (MRI)
    d. Keep the patient on a spine board until he recovers consciousness

44. **Which of the following statement regarding spine injury is *true*?**
    a. Cervical spine cord injuries are common
    b. The size of the spinal canal makes the cervical spine especially susceptible to injury
    c. The stability of the cervical spine is mainly provided by the bony anatomy
    d. The cervicothoracic junction is especially susceptible to injury because it is a transition zone from the mobile to the rigid segment of the spinal cord

45. **What organ is most at risk as the limbs start to reperfuse in a patient gradually rewarmed after a severe crush injury?**
    a. Brain—due to hypoxic shunting to the crushed limbs
    b. Liver—due to blood breakdown products
    c. Kidney—due to release of muscle degradation products
    d. Lung—due to multiple microemboli

46. **Neurological complications are common with COVID-19 infection. Which of the following is the least likely mechanism of SARS-CoV-2 causing neurological symptoms?**
    a. Entry of SARS-CoV-2 virus through the olfactory nerves
    b. Crosses the blood-brain barrier following viremia
    c. Entry via neuronal and mucosal alpha (α) receptors
    d. Innate adaptive immune response to the COVID-19 virus

47. **A 55-year-old man has quadriplegia after undergoing suboccipital craniotomy in the sitting position for the treatment of acoustic neuroma. Which of the following is the most likely cause?**
    a. Air embolism with the presence of probe patent foramen ovale
    b. Cervical cord compression
    c. Jugular venous obstruction
    d. Sustained elevation of CPP

48. **Which statement is *true* regarding analgesia and delirium?**
    a. Morphine is associated with increased incidence of delirium
    b. Patient controlled analgesia (PCA) use in contraindicated in patients with delirium
    c. Opioids should be avoided
    d. Inadequate analgesia may present similarly to delirium

49. **Which of the following is the most effective response to changes in body temperature?**
    a. Cutaneous vasoconstriction
    b. Cutaneous vasodilation
    c. Behavioral changes
    d. Non-shivering thermogenesis

50. **Regarding guidelines for brain death in children, which of the following is *true*?**
    a. Preterm infants less than 37 weeks gestational age are excluded from the guidelines
    b. Apnea testing is not required in children for diagnosing brain death
    c. EEG is mandatory in determining brain death in children
    d. One examination will suffice for determining brain death in children

51. **Which of the following is *true* regarding serum glucose in patients with injured brain?**
    a. Hypoglycemia has little impact on injured brain
    b. Hyperglycemia is not a problem in patients with cerebral ischemia
    c. Perioperative hyperglycemia is common in adults but not children undergoing craniotomy for traumatic brain injury
    d. Patients with intraoperative hyperglycemia during neurosurgical procedures are more likely to develop postoperative neurologic dysfunction

52. **A 54-year-old female with h/o severe aortic stenosis with moderate left ventricular failure, is scheduled for emergent craniotomy for evacuation of hematoma. Which of the following is *true*?**
    a. Rapid sequence induction with propofol is preferred
    b. Phenylephrine is preferred for treating hypotension
    c. Pulmonary catheter may not be valuable
    d. Mannitol is safe for brain relaxation for this patient

53. **During transsphenoidal pituitary surgery, which of the following is most appropriate?**
    a. Administer dexamethasone routinely for PONV prophylaxis
    b. Hyperventilate the patient to facilitate surgical exposure
    c. Tape the endotracheal tube at the upper lip close to midline
    d. Control blood pressure to reduce intraoperative nose bleeding

54. Which of the following statements concerning the cerebral effects of barbiturates is *true*?
    a. Barbiturate coma produces greater cerebral protection than hypothermia to 17°C
    b. Barbiturates decrease the cerebral metabolic rate for oxygen by decreasing CBF
    c. Somatosensory evoked potentials and the EEG are equally sensitive to suppression by barbiturates
    d. When administered in doses sufficient to produce an isoelectric EEG, barbiturates decrease the cerebral metabolic rate for oxygen by 50%

55. Regional cerebral metabolism is increased by:
    a. Halothane
    b. Mannitol
    c. Pain
    d. Ketamine

56. A 55-year-old patient undergoes elective craniotomy for tumor resection. How long prior to elective craniotomy should systemic steroids (methylprednisolone) be administered to show a reduction in edema formation, a reduction in ICP, and an improved clinical outcome?
    a. At least 6 hrs prior
    b. At least 12 hrs prior
    c. At least 24 hrs prior
    d. At least 48 hrs prior

57. Out of the following statements regarding osmotic agents to lower ICP, which statement is *incorrect*?
    a. They create an osmotic gradient forcing fluid into the intravascular compartment
    b. Mannitol and hypertonic saline (HTS) can cause hypernatremia
    c. In a situation of low blood pressure, mannitol is preferable
    d. Treatment goals for osmotic agents include serum osmolality 310–320 mOsm/L

58. A 39-year-old male presents with scoliosis for complex spine surgery. He is morbidly obese, diabetes, hypertensive. The surgery was prolonged with large volume blood loss. He was resuscitated with 7 L crystalloid, 6 packed cells, 3 FFP and 1 platelets for a 3.5 liter blood loss. 4 hours into the postoperative in the ICU, he had hypotension and difficulty with ventilation and oxygenation. CXR shows fluffy infiltrates. The following could be least likely diagnosis:
    a. Hemolytic transfusion reaction
    b. Adult respiratory distress syndrome
    c. Transfusion associated acute lung injury (TRALI)
    d. Transfusion associated circulatory overload (TACO)

59. A 49-year-old man was involved in a motor vehicle accident and was brought to the casualty with a cervical collar. On initial examination, he appears drowsy. He does not move all four extremities. His blood pressure is 88/48 and heart rate is 46. What is the reason for his shock?
    a. Vasodilation
    b. Cardiac failure
    c. Epinephrine release
    d. Blood loss

60. Which of the following is *incorrect* with respect to volatile anesthetics as a part of your anesthetic plan for neurosurgery?
    a. They make cerebral blood low pressure passive
    b. At 0.9 MAC, metabolic coupling is maintained
    c. They blunt the cerebrovascular response to CO_2
    d. Decreases $CMRO_2$ while increasing CBF

61. Which of the following will not alter the cerebral autoregulation?
    a. Hypercapnea
    b. Traumatic brain injury
    c. Propofol
    d. Volatile anesthetics in higher doses

62. Which maneuvre affects CBF the most?
    a. Change of PaO_2 from 120 to 70 mm Hg
    b. Change in MAC of isoflurane from 0.5 to 1.3
    c. Change in MAC of sevoflurane from 0.6 to 1.5
    d. Change of $PaCO_2$ from 40 to 60 mm Hg

63. Which of the following treatment for the traumatic spine injury is *incorrect*?
    a. Urinary catheterization
    b. Prevent hypotension
    c. Stress ulcer prophylaxis
    d. High dose steroids

64. A 65-year-old male with known history of deep vein thrombosis is on warfarin treatment. Patient has a fall and develops subdural hematoma requiring urgent exploration. Which treatment option is the least useful?
    a. Fresh frozen plasma
    b. Four factor prothrombin complex concentrate
    c. Oral vitamin K_1
    d. Recombinant Factor VIIa

65. Which of the following statements about pituitary adenomas is *false*?
    a. They most often arise from the anterior pituitary
    b. Functioning tumors produce a single, predominant hormone
    c. Micro-adenomas are usually nonfunctioning and detected incidentally
    d. Macro-adenomas present late with headache as the presenting complaint

66. Trans-sphenoidal approach for resection of pituitary tumor is NOT recommended for:
    a. Functioning pituitary adenoma
    b. Non-functioning adenoma
    c. Large pituitary adenoma
    d. Small pituitary adenoma

67. **Out of the following monitors which one is the least sensitive to detect venous air embolism?**
    a. Transesophageal echocardiogram
    b. ECG changes
    c. Capnography
    d. Pulmonary artery pressure

68. **About intraoperative evoked potential (EP) monitoring, which of the following statement is *true*?**
    a. Brainstem auditory EP (BAEP) are very sensitive to inhalational anesthetic agents
    b. 50% of nitrous oxide is acceptable to use during monitoring
    c. Midazolam and fentanyl have minimal effects on EP recordings
    d. Equipotent doses of inhalational and intravenous anesthetics suppress EP equally

69. **Regarding cerebral vasospasm which of the following statement is *incorrect*?**
    a. Vasospasm can be detected as early as in 3 hours of SAH
    b. Calcium channel blockers have a role in treatment of vasospasm
    c. Transcranial Doppler can show increase flow velocities before the actual ischemia setting in
    d. Endovascular therapy has no role in the treatment of vasospasm

70. **Which of the following is not *true* with regards to deep brain stimulator placement for Parkinson's disease?**
    a. Anti-Parkinson's medications should be given the morning of surgery
    b. The procedure is an awake surgery
    c. The lead is either placed at the subthalamic nucleus or the globus pallidus interna
    d. Uncontrolled dyskinesia is one of the primary indication of this surgery

71. **During a mechanical thrombectomy under monitored anesthesia care, a patient develops intracranial hematoma. Which maneuvre is *incorrect* from the following?**
    a. To maintain systolic blood pressure above 140 mm Hg
    b. Rapid lowering of blood pressure to prevent bleeding
    c. Should be converted to GA
    d. Intravenous Protamine should be given

72. **Which nerve is not anesthetized in the scalp block?**
    a. Supratrochlear nerve
    b. Lesser occipital nerve
    c. C4 cervical nerve root
    d. Branches of the ophthalmic division of the trigeminal nerve

73. **Which is not a characteristic feature of pituitary apoplexy?**
    a. 3rd cranial nerve palsy
    b. Severe headache
    c. Altered mental status
    d. Unilateral visual field defect

74. **What is not *true* about the brain metabolism?**
    a. Most of the transport of glucose in brain requires energy
    b. Ionic homeostasis in brain requires energy
    c. In hypoxemic conditions, anaerobic metabolism is insufficient for meeting brain energy requirements
    d. Glucose transport in brain is a passive process

75. **Which of the following does not cause hyperglycemia in traumatic brain injured patients?**
    a. Gluconeogenesis   b. Fentanyl
    c. Cortisol   d. Corticotropin

76. **What is not *true* about the trigeminal cardiac reflex (TCR)?**
    a. Can present as bradycardia and hypertension
    b. Hypocarbia is a precipitating factor
    c. Metoprolol can potentiate the reflex
    d. Can occur because of stimulation of either peripheral or central sections of trigeminal nerve

77. **Which of the following is *correct* for entropy - depth of anesthesia monitors?**
    a. Response entropy zero signifies awake state
    b. It uses SHANON equation
    c. It uses QUAZI analysis
    d. It uses 2 channels

78. **Match the *correct* EEG wave with their corresponding frequency:**

Wave	Frequency
A. Alpha	1. > 30 Hz
B. Beta	2. < 3 Hz
C. Delta	3. 13–30 Hz
D. Gamma	4. 7–12 Hz

    a. A-1, B-2, C-3, D-4
    b. A-3, B-1, C-4, D-2
    c. A-4, B-3, C-2, D-1
    d. A-2, B-4, C-1, D-3

79. **Isoelectric EEG is seen at what temperature?**
    a. 17ºC   b. 0ºC
    c. 27ºC   d. 37ºC

80. Which of the following is not *true* regarding as either prevention or the treatment of TCR?
    a. Regional anesthesia
    b. Adrenaline
    c. Preemptive atropine
    d. Clear communication with the surgeon

81. Which of the following statement is not *true* regarding coronary artery spasm during neurosurgical cases?
    a. Female gender is a risk factor
    b. It is a vagal mediated response
    c. It predominantly occurs in patients who have coronary artery disease
    d. Thalamic stimulation can precipitate the spasm

82. When is a pregnant woman with an intracranial arteriovenous malformation at greatest risk of rupture of the AVM?
    a. 1st trimester
    b. 2nd trimester
    c. 3rd trimester
    d. During labor

83. Spinal anesthesia for a cesarean section should be avoided in which of the parturients?
    a. A pregnant lady with intracranial aneurysm
    b. Parturients with tethered cord
    c. Parturients with pseudotumor cerebri
    d. None of the above parturients qualify

84. Which of the following about cerebral oximetry (near infrared spectroscopy) is *true*?
    a. It is a non-invasive measurement of regional cerebral oxygenation
    b. It measures the arterial oxygen in the brain
    c. The normal values are between 90 and 100
    d. It is more accurate when there is a component of extravascular blood

85. Which of the following is a *true* statement regarding pharmacological strategies in preventing postoperative delirium (POD)?
    a. Gabapentinoids increase the risk of POD
    b. Rivastigmine reduces the incidence of POD
    c. Diphenhydramine is useful in preventing POD
    d. Current evidence for antipsychotic prophylaxis for POD is insufficient

86. Which of the following statement for hepatic encephalopathy is not *correct*?
    a. Hypermagnesemia is one of the cause of encephalopathy
    b. Hypoxia can exacerbate the pre-existing cerebral edema
    c. Acute fulminant hepatic failure is a common cause of encephalopathy
    d. Ammonia causes astrocyte swelling

87. Which of the following agent does not contribute to neurodegeneration in neonates?
    a. Isoflurane
    b. Propofol
    c. Ketamine
    d. Dexmedetomidine

88. Which of the following is *true* regarding management of traumatic brain injury (TBI)?
    a. Glasgow Coma Scale can accurately predict the outcome after TBI
    b. Intracranial pressure monitoring can accurately predict the outcome following TBI
    c. The initial severity of the TBI will ultimately determine the final outcome
    d. Multimodal monitoring would better help to guide individual therapy following TBI

89. Which of the following statement regarding the pharmacokinetics of ketamine is *incorrect*?
    a. It is highly lipid soluble
    b. The elimination half life is 2–3 hours
    c. Metabolized by liver
    d. The bioavailability of intranasal route is 90%

90. Which of the following is *incorrect* for hyperventilation as a method to reduce the ICP?
    a. It takes 2 hours for hyperventilation to become clinically effective
    b. If hyperventilation is stopped abruptly, it can result in rebound cerebral edema
    c. Cerebral ischemia is known complication of hyperventilation
    d. The effect of hyperventilation lasts for approximately 8 hours

91. A surgeon is operating a pineal gland glioma in sitting position. During craniotomy there is sudden hypotension, tachycardia with fall of $ETCO_2$ from 35 mm Hg to 16 mm Hg. Which of the following is the *incorrect* step in the management?
    a. Flushing the field with saline
    b. Reverse Trendelenburg position
    c. Aspiration of the central venous catheter
    d. Fluid bolus

92. During an aneurysmal clipping surgery, there is a sudden intraoperative rupture of aneurysm. Which of the following is NOT a treatment option in emergent management?
    a. Blood transfusion
    b. Propofol bolus
    c. Induced hypothermia
    d. Cardiac arrest with adenosine

93. Which of the statements about postoperative visual loss (POVL) after spine surgery is *false*?
    a. Ischemic optic neuropathy (ION) is associated with emboli into the retinal artery
    b. A central retinal artery occlusion (CRAO) is usually unilateral
    c. ION is the most common cause for permanent POVL
    d. Central retinal artery occlusion is associated with direct compression of the globe

94. Which of the following statements about ICP is *true*?
    a. ICP should be maintained below 30 mm Hg
    b. In a patient with severe TBI with a normal CT scan, ICP monitor can be excluded
    c. ICP measurement is the direct reflection of CBF
    d. Hyperventilation for raised ICP should only be used for a brief period

95. Which cells in cerebral cortex are responsible for EEG generation?
    a. Golgi cells
    b. Pyramidal cells
    c. Stellate cells
    d. Glial cells

96. Zipper opening pattern (EEG signatures) signifies which of the following feature of anesthesia?
    a. Induction of anesthesia with propofol
    b. Ketamine sedation
    c. Maintenance of anesthesia with inhalational anesthesia
    d. Awakening of anesthesia

97. Burst suppression is seen in which form of EEG analysis?
    a. Time domain analysis
    b. Phase domain analysis
    c. Frequency domain analysis
    d. Amplitude domain analysis

98. Which one of the following is measured by near infrared spectroscopy?
    a. Non-invasive, global oxygenation
    b. Invasive, focal oxygenation
    c. Invasive global oxygenation
    d. Non-invasive focal oxygenation

99. What arterial to venous ratio of contribution is incorporated in near infrared spectroscopy technology?
    a. 25 : 75
    b. 50 : 50
    c. 40 : 60
    d. 30 : 70

100. Transcranial Doppler measures:
    a. Blood volume in brain circulation
    b. Blood pressure in brain circulation
    c. Blood flow velocity in brain circulation
    d. Blood vessel diameter in brain circulation

101. Frequency of ultrasound probe sued for transcranial Doppler is:
    a. 2 MHz
    b. 5 MHz
    c. 10 MHz
    d. 8 MHz

102. Gold standard for ICP monitoring is:
    a. Intra-parenchymal catheter
    b. Subdural catheter
    c. Intra-ventricular catheter
    d. Epidural catheter

103. Which of the following is not a grading system used in SAH?
    a. WFNS
    b. Modified Fischer grade
    c. Hunt and Hess grade
    d. Marshall's grade

104. Antagonist of rivaroxaban is:
    a. Idarucizumab
    b. Andexanet alfa
    c. Fresh frozen plasma
    d. Vitamin K

105. Which anatomical site is described by Dennis three column model?
    a. Spinal cord
    b. Brain
    c. Vertebral column
    d. Vascular system

106. CRASH-3 trial is associated with which drug?
    a. Tranexamic acid
    b. Methylprednisolone
    c. Dexamethasone
    d. Ondansetron

107. Which is not included in the concept of triple low in anesthesia practice?
    a. MAC < 0.7
    b. MAP < 75 mm Hg
    c. BIS < 45
    d. Entropy < 50

108. Dexamethasone is used to reduce:
    a. Interstitial edema
    b. Cytotoxic edema
    c. Vasogenic edema
    d. Osmotic edema

109. Pupillary dilatation in severe traumatic brain injury patients is due to the:
    a. 3rd nerve compression
    b. Herniation of tonsils
    c. Herniation of lateral temporal lobe
    d. Hyperoxia

110. Which of the following is not *correct* about postoperative visual loss?
    a. It is a rare complication
    b. Mostly seen with prone craniotomy
    c. Hypotension, hemodilution and prolonged surgery are important risk factors
    d. Cherry red macula is seen in ION

111. Sodium content of Plasma-lyte A intravenous fluid is:
    a. 26 mEq/L
    b. 52 mEq/L
    c. 90 mEq/L
    d. 140 mEq/L

112. **Rivaroxaban, a non-vitamin K antagonist oral anticoagulants (NOACs) acts by inhibition of:**
    a. Factor XI a
    b. Factor X a
    c. Factor X a and II a
    d. Factor II a

113. **Which of the following trials evaluated role of corticosteroid in patients with TBI?**
    a. ENIGMA
    b. IMPACT
    c. DECRA
    d. CRASH

114. **Atlantoaxial dislocation in adult is defined as:**
    a. Anterior atlantodental interval (ADI) greater than 5 mm
    b. ADI greater 3 mm
    c. PDI (posterior atlantodental interval) greater 3 mm
    d. PDI less than 5 mm

115. **All of the following regarding myasthenia gravis is true, except:**
    a. Ice-pack test can be used for diagnosis
    b. More common in males
    c. It requires immunosuppression
    d. Some cases need plasmapheresis

116. **Which of the following is false regarding surface tension in an alveolus?**
    a. Smaller alveoli tend to empty into larger ones
    b. Dipalmitoylphosphatidyl choline reduces surface tension
    c. Surfactant is secreted by type IV pneumocytes
    d. Positive end-expiratory pressure (PEEP) counteracts surface tension

117. **Which of the following are identified as lactose fermenting bacteria on MacConkey medium?**
    a. *Escherichia coli, Enterobacteria*
    b. *Salmonella, Proteus, Yersinia*
    c. *Staphylococci*
    d. *Acid fast bacilli*

118. **Which of the following is false regarding emphysema of lungs?**
    a. Diffusing capacity for carbon monoxide is reduced
    b. Residual lung volume is increased
    c. Lung compliance is decreased
    d. Is commonly associated with smoking and chronic obstructive pulmonary disease (COPD)

119. **Which of the following is true regarding extended-spectrum beta-lactamases (ESBL) producing organisms?**
    a. They are gram-positive organisms
    b. They are resistant to cephamycins like cefoxitin, cefotetan
    c. They are resistant to fourth generation cephalosporins like cefepime
    d. They are intrinsically resistant to carbapenems

120. **Which of the following is false regarding functional residual capacity (FRC)**
    a. It is determined by the balance between elastic recoil of lung and chestwall.
    b. It helps in preventing desaturation after exhalation.
    c. Lung compliance would decrease in absence of FRC
    d. Continuous positive airway pressure (CPAP) therapy reduces FRC

121. **A 62-year-old male underwent CABG and is being monitored in ICU. Four hours postoperatively, suddenly, the monitor shows the below pattern on ECG. Next best step in management would be:**
    a. IV Adrenaline
    b. IV Adenosine
    c. Defibrillation
    d. Check pulse and blood pressure

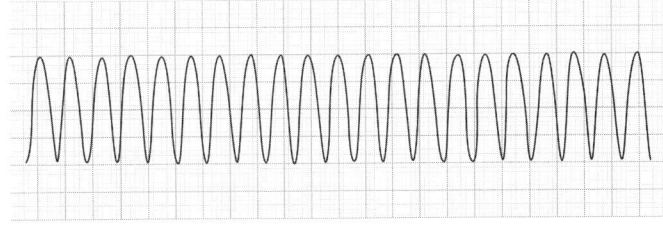

122. **High quality CPR for adult victim contains all except:**
    a. Chest compressions of at least 2 inches
    b. Minimizing interruptions between compressions
    c. Change of compressor every 5 minutes of compressions
    d. 30:2 compression – ventilation ratio

123. **In invasive arterial BP monitoring, square wave test is showing more than 2 oscillations when returning to baseline, and your arterial pressure waveform has an exaggerated appearance. What does that infer?**
    a. Optimally damped
    b. Overdamped system
    c. Underdamped system
    d. Loose fitting of the tubing

124. **Following is true with regards to electrical safety and prevention of explosions:**
    a. Nitrous oxide is not flammable at atmospheric pressure
    b. Anesthetic machines should be isolated from 'earth' to prevent completion of an electrical circuit
    c. Currents of 10 microamps may initiate ventricular fibrillation
    d. In surgical diathermy the heat released depends on the square of the potential difference between electrodes

125. **Regarding ulnar neuropathy related to intraoperative positioning under anesthesia, which is incorrect?**

a. Is the most common perioperative neuropathy
b. 80% of 'only sensory neuropathy' resolve within 6 months
c. 20% of the combined sensory-motor neuropathy result in permanent motor dysfunction and pain
d. 80% of the combined sensory-motor neuropathy result in permanent motor dysfunction and pain

126. **Choose the *correct* option for this mainstream capnography waveform:**

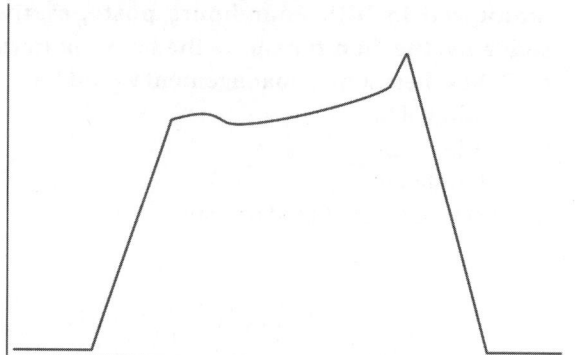

a. Abnormal waveform seen in thin individuals with normal lungs
b. Normal waveform seen in lungs with good compliance
c. Normal waveform seen in very early pregnancy
d. Normal waveform seen in advanced pregnancy

127. **Following changes in the coagulation system are seen in normal pregnancy:**
a. All pro-coagulants increase and platelets decrease
b. Factors XI, XIII, antithrombin III, protein S, platelets decrease while II, V, protein C levels remain unchanged
c. Marked increase in factor I and factor VII with 20% increase in prothrombin time
d. Increase in I, VII, VIII, IX, X, XII von Willebrand factor and anticoagulant factors

128. **Dural puncture epidural technique for labor analgesia is:**
a. Another name for CSE technique
b. Placement of epidural catheter through inadvertent dural puncture
c. Dural puncture with 25 gauge spinal needle using "needle-through-needle" technique after locating epidural with epidural needle with no medication into the intrathecal space
d. Sequential subarachnoid/epidural technique of injecting opioid followed by local anesthetic

129. **As per the 2020 AHA ACLS algorithm for cardiac arrest in in-hospital pregnant patients, in the potential etiology as per A, B, C, D, E, F, G, H mnemonic, H stands for:**
a. Hypotension
b. Hypertension
c. Hyperemesis gravidarum
d. Hypothyroidism

130. **With regard to cardiovascular changes in normal pregnancy, when does the cardiac output returns to prepregnancy levels?**
a. Immediately postpartum
b. 6 – 8 weeks postpartum
c. 8 – 10 weeks postpartum
d. 12 – 24 weeks postpartum

131. **With regard to respiratory changes, third trimester in normal pregnancy is characterized by:**
a. Increased PaO_2, $PaCO_2$, HCO_3 and pH
b. Decreased PaO_2, $PaCO_2$, HCO_3 and pH
c. Increased PaO_2, decreased $PaCO_2$ and HCO_3 with pH towards alkalotic side
d. Decreased PaO_2, $PaCO_2$, HCO_3 and pH of 7.4

132. **Changes in sleep pattern in normal pregnancy is characterized by:**
a. Increased sleep time, decreased stage 3 and 4 NREM in 1st trimester with decreased REM and total sleep in 3rd trimester
b. Increased sleep time, increased stage 3 and 4 NREM from 1st to 3rd trimester
c. Decreased sleep time, decreased stage 3 and 4 NREM, increased REM from 1st to 3rd trimester
d. Decreased sleep time, increased stage 3 and 4 NREM in 1st trimester and increased sleep and REM in 3rd trimester leading to OSA in late pregnancy

133. **Appropriate cricoid pressure in pregnancy is achieved by applying:**
a. Initial force of 20 N when patient is awake increased to 40 N as patient becomes unconscious
b. A steady force of 30 N throughout the intubation attempt
c. Initial force of 10 N when patient is awake increased to 30 N as patient becomes unconscious
d. Initial force of 20 N when patient is awake increased to 45 N as patient becomes unconscious

134. **Select the drugs that readily cross placental barrier:**
a. Succinylcholine, vecuronium, pancuronium
b. Atropine, glycopyrrolate
c. Propofol, thiopentone, ketamine
d. Ephedrine, phenylephrine, nitroglycerin

135. **Choice of drug to treat bradycardia during neonatal resuscitation:**
a. Glycopyrrolate   b. Atropine
c. Ephedrine   d. Epinephrine

136. **Recommended dose of 20% lipid emulsion in treatment of local anesthetic systemic toxicity is:**
    a. 1.5 mg/kg bolus followed by 0.25 mg/kg infusion not exceeding 10 mg/kg in 30 minutes
    b. 1.5 mL/kg bolus followed by 0.25 mL/kg/hr infusion not exceeding 12 mL/kg
    c. 1.5 mL/kg bolus followed by 0.25 mL/kg/min infusion not exceeding 12 mL/kg
    d. 1.5 mg/kg bolus followed by 0.25 mg/kg/min infusion not exceeding 10 mg/kg in 30 minutes

137. **ACLS in treatment of local anesthetic systemic toxicity in pregnancy involves:**
    a. Epinephrine in higher doses than normal and use of vasopressin
    b. Epinephrine in lower doses than normal and use of vasopressin
    c. Epinephrine in higher doses than normal and avoiding vasopressin
    d. Epinephrine in lower doses than normal and avoiding vasopressin

138. **Following features were seen after catheter placement and approximately 15 minutes after injection of local anesthetic for labor analgesia, cranial nerve involvement with no sacral analgesia, patchy block, inability to speak, 10–20 mm Hg drop in systolic blood pressure. This is suggestive of catheter placement in:**
    a. Intrathecal space with total spinal anesthesia
    b. Intrathecal space with high spinal anesthesia
    c. Epidural space
    d. Subdural space

139. **In patients administered epidural analgesia for labor, second stage arrest is defined by no progress (descent or rotation) for:**
    a. Four hours or more in nulliparous women, 3 hours or more in parous women
    b. Five hours or more nulliparous women, 3 hours or more in parous women
    c. Four hours or more in nulliparous women, 2 hours or more in parous women
    d. Six hours or more in nulliparous women, 4 hours or more in parous women

140. **Following technique was used in a patient posted for Category 1 caesarean section-informed consent, intravenous line secured by staff, preoxygenation, 'No Touch Technique', donning only gloves, chlorhexidine painting, using glove packet as sterile surface, single attempt spinal with 2.8 cc bupivacaine (heavy), surgery started once sensory level >T10 and ascending with general anesthesia readiness. The technique best represents:**
    a. Routine subarachnoid block for Category 1 caesarean section
    b. Low resource technique for Category 1 caesarean section
    c. Rapid sequence spinal for Category 1 caesarean section
    d. Double setup technique for Category 1 caesarean section

141. **Following drug is preferred in treatment of spinal hypotension during caeserean section in patients with gestational hypertension:**
    a. Phenylephrine or ephedrine
    b. Phenylephrine or mephentermine
    c. Ephedrine or mephentermine
    d. Mephentermine

142. **Which of the following statement is *false* regarding use of phenylephrine for treatment of spinal hypotension in pregnant patients?**
    a. Higher doses are required for treatment as compared to non-pregnant patients
    b. Phenylephrine has decreased uterine vascular resistance as compared to ephedrine
    c. Placental transfer is greater for ephedrine than phenylephrine, with less early metabolism and/or redistribution in the fetus
    d. Administration of atropine to treat reflex bradycardia can result in significant hypertensive response

143. **Which of the following statement is *false* with respect to use of patient controlled analgesia (PCA) for post caesarean pain relief?**
    a. During PCA, a high ratio of patient demands to delivered bolus doses, signifies adequate pain relief
    b. PCA can be used via the intravenous and epidural routes
    c. Programmable PCA parameters include drug choice, bolus dose, maximum dose, and lockout interval
    d. Use of opioids should invoke the application of algorithms for pain assessment, management, and monitoring

144. **Which of the following statement is *correct* with respect to timing of epidural catheter placement and intravascular balloon catheter for obstetric hemorrhage?**
    a. Once the balloon catheter is placed, flexion of the hips during positioning for a neuraxial anesthetic technique is discouraged, because it may result in balloon dislodgement or occlusion and subsequent thrombosis
    b. Use of local anesthesia with sedation for balloon catheter placement is preferable than epidural analgesia

c. Epidural catheter if needed should be preferably placed after balloon catheter placement
d. Epidural catheter should not be used for cesarean delivery as heparin is given during the procedure

145. Which of the following statement is *false* with respect to use of opioids for postcaesarean pain relief?
    a. Meperidine is recommended in obstetric patients due to longer duration of action and no effect on fetus
    b. A 25-μg/h transdermal fentanyl patch is equianalgesic to approximately 50 mg of oral morphine per day
    c. Morphine is relatively contraindicated in patients with impaired renal function
    d. Intrathecal morphine 0.075 – 0.2 mg is equivalent to epidural morphine 2 – 3 mg

146. Which of the following definitions is an *incorrect* match?
    a. Gestational hypertension: 20 weeks gestational age to 12 weeks postpartum, proteinuria present
    b. Preeclampsia: 20 weeks gestational age to 12 weeks postpartum, proteinuria present
    c. Chronic hypertension: Prior to 20 weeks gestational age and lasts beyond 12 weeks postpartum
    d. Severe preeclampsia: 20 weeks gestational age to 12 weeks postpartum, BP >160/110, proteinuria 2+ present, persistent headache, S. Creatinine >1.2 mg%, persistent epigastric pain, platelets <1 lakh/cu mm

147. Which of the following is *true* about gestational diabetes mellitus?
    a. Maternal insulin requirements decrease with the onset of labor, increase again during the second stage of labor
    b. Intravenous glucose and insulin infusions during the peripartum period should be titrated to maintain a maternal blood glucose concentration of 110–140 L to prevent neonatal hypoglycemia
    c. Diabetic scleredema can lead to increased local anesthetic volume requirement during neuraxial anesthesia
    d. Pregnancy may accelerate the progression of diabetic nephropathy, but not proliferative retinopathy

148. Which of the following is *false* about neuraxial opioid induced respiratory depression?
    a. Respiratory monitoring after neuraxial administration of morphine should occur at least every hour for the first 12 hours and then every 2 hours for the next 12 hours
    b. Respiratory monitoring after administration of neuraxial fentanyl should continue for a minimum of 2 hours
    c. Early-onset respiratory depression associated with lipophilic opioids usually occurs within 30 minutes of administration
    d. As per recent studies respiratory depression after neuraxial morphine administration is triphasic-immediate dose dependent, delayed due to rostral spread, late onset during dissociation phase

149. Which of the following is *false* about neuraxial opioid induced pruritus?
    a. Opioid-induced histamine release from mast cells appears to be one of the causative mechanism for pruritus after neuraxial opioid administration
    b. Pregnant patients may be more susceptible as a result of estrogen interaction with opioid receptors
    c. There may be a genetic predisposition to pruritus due to opioid receptor genotype
    d. Pentazocine, a κ-opioid receptor agonist and partial μ-opioid receptor agonist, may be a useful drug for treating opioid-induced pruritus

150. Select the *incorrect* pair of uterotonic drugs to relative contraindications and/or extreme caution during administration:
    a. Carboprost: Asthma
    b. Misoprostol: Malignant hyperthermia
    c. Oxytocin: Malignant hyperthermia
    d. Methylergonovine: Gestational hypertension

151. Which of the following is *false* about placental transfer of drugs?
    a. Dantrolene crosses the placenta and may result in neonatal hypotonia if administered before delivery
    b. Dabigatran crosses the placenta with an F/M ratio of 0.33
    c. Sodium nitroprusside is lipid soluble, rapidly crosses the placenta, and can produce cyanide as a byproduct
    d. Sugammadex, unlike neuromuscular blocking agents, has high placental transfer rates

152. Match the needles:

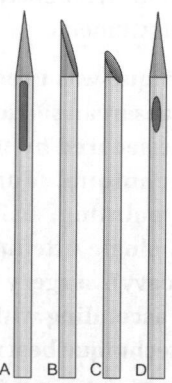

a. A-SPROTTE, B-WHITACRE, C-QUINCKE, D-PITKIN
b. A-WHITACRE, B-QUINCKE, C-SPROTTE, D-PITKIN
c. A-WHITACRE, B-QUINCKE, C-PITKIN, D-SPROTTE
d. A-SPROTTE, B-QUINCKE, C-PITKIN, D-WHITACRE

153. **Which of the following is *false* about the following tocolytic drugs?**
    a. Atosiban used in Europe has been associated with a few perinatal deaths
    b. Nifedipine to be used with care with volatile halogenated anesthetic agents
    c. Indomethacin causes maternal platelet dysfunction and so is a contraindication for neuraxial anesthesia
    d. Terbutaline can cause hypotension, tachycardia, cardiac arrhythmias and myocardial ischemia, pulmonary edema, hyperglycemia and hypokalemia

154. **Which of the following is *false* about the posterior reversible leukoencephalopathy syndrome (PRES)?**
    a. Conditions associated with PRES include preeclampsia, uremia, hemolytic-uremic syndrome, infection, malignancy, and COVID-19
    b. Symptoms include headache, seizures, altered mental status, visual changes, and, occasionally, focal neurologic deficits
    c. As the name suggests, it is always reversible with treatment
    d. MRI is gold standard for early diagnosis

155. **Which of the following is not a known differential diagnosis of postpartum headache?**
    a. Posterior reversible leukoencephalopathy syndrome
    b. Postdural puncture headache
    c. Ondansetron headache
    d. Paradoxical oxytocin headache

156. **Which of the following is a hallmark of peripartum cardiomyopathy?**
    a. Onset of heart failure during the last month of pregnancy or within 5 months of delivery with no other identifiable cause of heart failure and no known heart disease before pregnancy
    b. Onset of heart failure anytime during pregnancy with no other identifiable cause of heart failure and no known heart disease before pregnancy
    c. Pregnancy associated dynamic left ventricular outflow tract obstruction with obstruction gradient typically increasing after a premature ventricular contraction
    d. Potentially reversible condition during labor associated with rapid atrial or ventricular rates caused by arrhythmias in pregnancy

157. **Match the following doses of anti-hypertensive agents:**
    1. Labetalol   A. 5 mg IV every 20 min up to 20 mg IV
    2. Hydralazine B. 5 mg/h, increase by 2.5 mg/h every 5 min to 15 mg/h
    3. Nifedipine   C. 20 mg IV, then 40–80 mg every 10 min up to 220 mg
    4. Nicardipine D. 10 mg PO every 20 min up to 50 mg

    a. 1-A, 2-D, 3-B, 4-C
    b. 1-B, 2-C, 3-A, 4-D
    c. 1-D, 2-C, 3-A, 4-B
    d. 1-C, 2-A, 3-D, 4-B

158. **Which of the following is not a known WHO recommendation for oxytocin?**
    a. Oxytocin does not require cold chain, hence recommended in low resource setups
    b. Umbilical vein injection of oxytocin is recommended for the treatment of retained placenta only in the context of rigorous research
    c. 10 IU oxytocin intramuscular/intravenous is recommended for the prevention of postpartum hemorrhage for all births
    d. Fixed-dose combination of oxytocin and ergometrine (5 IU/500 µg, IM) is recommended for the prevention of PPH in contexts where hypertensive disorders can be safely excluded prior to its use.

159. **Which of the following is *false* about anti-hypertensive drugs used in hypertensive disorders of pregnancy?**
    a. Labetalol should be avoided in women with severe asthma or congestive heart failure
    b. Hydralazine has side effects of maternal hypotension, tachycardia, palpitations, headache, and neonatal thrombocytopenia
    c. Nicardipine is now recommended as a first-line agent in women for whom intravenous access is difficult to secure
    d. Neonates born to mothers exposed to labetalol during delivery demonstrate increased rates of neonatal hypoglycemia and bradycardia

160. **Which of the following is *false* about cardiopulmonary bypass during pregnancy?**
    a. The degree of hypothermia is associated with poor fetal outcome
    b. The need for intraoperative fetal heart rate monitoring is universally accepted
    c. Measures to lower fetal mortality include hypothermic cardiopulmonary bypass with flow rates >2.4 L/min/m^2 while maintaining mean arterial blood pressure above 70–75 mm Hg
    d. Left uterine displacement and maintenance of a hematocrit greater than 28% are recommended

161. Select the *correct* statement with respect to eclampsia:
    a. Eclampsia is absolute contraindication for neuraxial anesthesia
    b. Magnesium sulfate is preferred to diazepam for the prevention of further seizures in eclampsia
    c. Fetal bradycardia typically begins during or immediately after a seizure and mandates immediate delivery
    d. Late eclampsia is defined as seizure onset from 24 hours after delivery to 6 weeks postpartum

162. Which of the following is *false* for treatment of uterine atony?
    a. Exogenous oxytocin can cause vasodilation, tachycardia, hypotension, coronary vasoconstriction, myocardial ischemia, and, rarely, even death, especially in hypovolemic or hemodynamically compromised women
    b. High doses of oxytocin administered concomitantly with large volumes of intravenous fluids, especially those containing free water, can lead to hyponatremia, seizures, and coma
    c. Carbetocin has a longer duration of action than oxytocin, eliminating the need for prolonged infusion
    d. ED 90 is almost ten times lower, approximately 3 IU, in women undergoing cesarean delivery for labor arrest after labor augmentation or induction with oxytocin

163. A parturient had a prolonged second stage of labor. Post-delivery she complained of difficulty in climbing stairs with no difficulty while walking on level ground. Which is the nerve most likely involved?
    a. Obturator nerve
    b. Sciatic nerve
    c. Common peroneal nerve
    d. Femoral nerve

164. Which of the following is *false* about the following blood and blood products?
    a. The concentration of citrate is seven times higher in fresh frozen plasma (FFP) and platelets than in PRBCs
    b. Whole blood is associated with lower rates of acute tubular necrosis
    c. Bacterial contamination occasionally occurs, most often during platelet transfusion
    d. If the blood type is unknown and blood products are required immediately, type O Rh positive RBCs and type AB plasma can be administered to obstetric patients

165. Which of the following is *false* about role of tranexamic acid in PPH?
    a. Administration beyond 3 hours does not confer clinical benefit
    b. If cryoprecipitate is not available, tranexamic acid 1 gram intravenously may be administered
    c. Tranexamic acid crosses the placenta
    d. Not to exceed 1 g administered slowly over 10 minutes; repeated once if bleeding continues after 30 minutes, followed by continuous infusion

166. Regarding near infrared spectroscopy (NIRS), the following statement is *incorrect*:
    a. It measures cerebral regional oxygen saturation
    b. Clinically important when decreases more than 20% from baseline
    c. Detects imbalance between oxygen supply and demand
    d. Normal value is always above 75%

167. Apgar score in neonates includes all, *except*:
    a. Heart rate
    b. Respiratory rate
    c. Muscle tone
    d. Color

168. Which of the following regarding neurotoxicity and general anesthetics is NOT *true*?
    a. All anesthetic agents that are NMDA antagonists or GABA agonists are associated with long lasting neurodevelopmental defects in experimental nonhuman studies
    b. Multiple exposures rather than one single exposure predispose to adverse neurodevelopmental outcome
    c. The MASK study has shown that in children less than 3 years exposed to general anesthetic did not have a decrease in general intelligence
    d. Multiply exposed children did not show a decrease in motor skills, behavioral speed, processing and reading

169. The cricoid ring is located at which level at birth?
    a. C3   b. C4
    c. C5   d. C6

170. Which of the following is not a part of difficult airway algorithm in pediatrics?
    a. Optimize head position
    b. Insert oral airway
    c. Percutaneous tracheostomy
    d. Cricothyroidotomy

171. Regarding EXIT procedure, which of the following statements is *FALSE*?
    a. It is important to maintain uterine relaxation

b. Uterine incision to cord-clamping interval should not exceed 3 minutes
c. Anesthetic agents given to the mother will cross the placental barrier
d. The major indication for this procedure is the need to secure the baby's airway before cord-clamping

172. **With respect to the transitional circulation in the newborn, which statement is *true*?**
    a. Expansion of the lungs at birth causes pulmonary vascular resistance to decrease dramatically to adult levels
    b. The transition from fetal to adult circulation is complete at the time of birth
    c. Fetal circulation is two circuits in parallel while adult circulation is in series
    d. NSAIDs such as indomethacin cause a patent ductus arteriosus to stay open

173. **With respect to an inhaled foreign body, choose the most appropriate statement:**
    a. Will be visible on the chest X-ray
    b. Fasting guidelines should be followed if the child is stable
    c. Decreased air entry with hyperinflated lung fields on that side is inconsistent with a foreign body bronchus
    d. Bronchoscopy is not considered an aerosol generating procedure

174. **For cleft lip surgery, these are the components of the "rule of 10's":**
    a. Weight 10 lbs, age 10 months, hematocrit 10%
    b. Weight 10 kg, age 10 weeks, Hb 10 gm/dL
    c. Weight 10 lbs, age 10 months, Hb 10 gm/dL
    d. Weight 10 lbs, age 10 weeks, Hb 10 gm/dL

175. **Regarding obstructive sleep apnea in children, the following statements are *true, except*:**
    a. The peak age for OSA in children is from 2 to 6 years of age
    b. Ventilatory response to CO_2 is attenuated
    c. Young children with OSA are generally obese
    d. Overnight pulse oximetry is a good indicator of severity of OSA

176. **The energy for defibrillation during CPR in a child is:**
    a. 2–4 J/kg
    b. 6–8 J/kg
    c. 10–12 J/kg
    c. None of the above

177. **All of the following are *true* about malignant hyperthermia (MH), *except*:**
    a. The earliest clinical sign is increase in end tidal CO_2
    b. Cola-colored urine is a late sign
    c. All inhalational anesthetics can trigger MH, *except* xenon
    d. Loading dose of dantrolene for treatment is 1 mg/kg

178. **Which of the following is *true* about emergence delirium (ED) in children?**
    a. The incidence is least in children 1–5 years of age
    b. The threshold PAED score to diagnose ED is ≥10
    c. The incidence is less with sevoflurane compared to desflurane
    d. The incidence after inhalational anesthesia is <1%

179. **Clear fluids are emptied from the stomach with a half-life of approximately:**
    a. 10 minutes
    b. 20 minutes
    c. 60 minutes
    d. 90 minutes

180. **The rapid increase of FA/FI (alveolar concentration/inspired concentration) of inhalational anesthetics in neonates is due to:**
    a. Higher functional residual capacity
    b. Reduced tissue/gas solubility in the vessel rich group of tissues
    c. Reduced alveolar ventilation
    d. None of the above

181. **All of the following about local anesthetics are *true, except*:**
    a. Dose of amide local anesthetics should be decreased by 30% in infants younger than 6 months of age
    b. The initial dose of intralipid to treat local anesthetic systemic toxicity is 1 mL/kg of 20% intralipid
    c. Greatest uptake (blood concentration) is with intercostal block
    d. Neurological features precede cardiovascular collapse

182. **Regarding eye surgery in children, which of these statements is *true*?**
    a. Oculocardiac reflex cannot be prevented by peribulbar block
    b. Strabismus is thought to increase chances of malignant hyperthermia
    c. Succinylcholine is contraindicated because it increases intraocular pressure
    d. Coughing during open eye surgery can cause prolapse of intraocular contents

183. **Regarding regional blocks in children, which of these statements is *false*?**
    a. Pediatric Regional Anesthesia Network database showed that regional blocks performed under

general anesthesia were associated with no incidence of permanent neurological deficits
b. Breakthrough pain from a working regional block, increased agitation and anxiety may indicate the onset of compartment syndrome in a child with limb fracture
c. Wake-up test during scoliosis surgery is contraindicated in children
d. The cardiovascular collapse/CNS (CC/CNS) ratio is "the ratio of drug dose required to cause catastrophic cardiovascular collapse to the drug dose required to produce seizures"

184. **Regarding burns in children, identify the *true* statement:**
    a. Succinylcholine is contraindicated within the first 24 hours after a major burn
    b. Facial burns are a warning of possible airway burns and inhalational injury
    c. Wallace rule of nines is used to estimate percent of burnt body surface area, similar to adults
    d. Parkland formula for fluid resuscitation is not used in children

185. **Regarding the use of theophylline which statement is *incorrect*?**
    a. The medication has a narrow therapeutic range
    b. It inhibits phosphodiesterase and is an adenosine receptor antagonist
    c. It is not effective orally
    d. Side effects include sleep disturbances, nausea, vomiting, and headaches

186. **Regarding intussusception, the following statement is NOT *true*:**
    a. Has a peak incidence in infants less than 1 year of age
    b. Presents with colicky abdominal pain, bloody (currant jelly) stools and vomiting
    c. May be reduced with a carefully performed enema
    d. Is nearly always caused by a "lead point" such as a polyp or duplication

187. **Regarding duodenal atresia, the following statement is *false*:**
    a. Often presents with vomiting which may or may not be bilious
    b. Radiography shows double bubble appearance
    c. Is associated with midline defects viz. esophageal atresia and imperforate anus
    d. Generally does not present until 1–2 months of life

188. **Regarding infantile hypertrophic pyloric stenosis, the following statement is NOT *true*:**
    a. The child develops metabolic alkalosis due to vomiting of gastric contents
    b. These infants are at increased risk of postoperative apnea
    c. Hyperkalemia and metabolic acidosis may be a feature
    d. The diagnosis is best made with a barium swallow

189. **The degree of shunting in a left-to-right shunt is significantly affected by all these factors, *except*:**
    a. Size of the defect
    b. Contractility of the heart
    c. Ratio of pulmonary vascular resistance to systemic vascular resistance
    d. Blood viscosity

190. **In the preoperative optimization of a child scheduled for pheochromocytoma excision, which of the following statements is *false*?**
    a. Unopposed beta stimulation following alpha adrenergic blockade can cause tachycardia and arrhythmias
    b. Phenoxybenzamine is a non-selective, non-competitive alpha blocker
    c. Patients are generally intravascular volume depleted
    d. It is important to initiate beta blocker therapy before alpha blocker therapy to prevent side effects

191. **With respect to left ventricular outflow tract obstruction which of the following statements is *true*?**
    a. ECMO has no role following cardiac arrest in patients due to outflow tract obstruction
    b. Avoid decrease in systemic vascular resistance and fast heart rate
    c. Pulmonary vascular resistance and systemic vascular resistance have little anesthetic concerns
    d. Etiology of most cardiac arrests in this group of patients is pulmonary artery hypertension

192. **Compared with normal adults, which of the following characteristics of neonates BEST explains the more rapid inhalation induction in neonates?**
    a. Greater cardiac index
    b. Greater metabolic rate
    c. Greater perfusion of vessel-rich tissues
    d. Greater ratio of alveolar ventilation to functional residual capacity

193. **Regarding caudal block in infants, the following statement is *true*:**
    a. Caudal administration of 0.25% bupivacaine will provide analgesia without evidence of motor block

b. Caudal administration of 0.125% bupivacaine is as effective as caudal administration of 0.25% bupivacaine
c. Caudal analgesia is more difficult to achieve in young children than in adults
d. The recommended volume of local anesthetic used for caudal analgesia in children is 3 mL per year of age

194. Which of the following features is characteristic of the airway in a neonate?
    a. Glottis that is located at the level of the C6 vertebral body
    b. Larger tongue relative to the oropharynx than in an adult
    c. Laryngeal mucosa that is densely adherent to the cartilages
    d. More posterior glottis than that of an adult

195. During Harrington rod instrumentation for scoliosis, monitoring somatosensory evoked potentials, the following statement is *true*:
    a. Is unreliable if halothane is used
    b. Eliminates the need for a wake-up test
    c. Accurately assesses proprioceptive integrity
    d. Accurately assesses motor function integrity

196. Which of the following statements concerning caudal anesthesia in children is *true*?
    a. The dural sac extends further caudad than in adults
    b. Delay of postoperative micturition occurs in most patients
    c. The sensory level of analgesia is poorly correlated with the dose of local anesthetic
    d. It is technically difficult because of poorly defined sacral anatomy

197. A 10-week-old infant born at 28 weeks gestation is scheduled for elective repair of bilateral inguinal hernia. It is most appropriate to:
    a. Delay the operation until the infant is 6 months old
    b. Transfuse blood preoperatively if hemoglobin concentration is 9 g/dL
    c. Avoid tracheal intubation
    d. Monitor for apnea for 24 hours postoperatively

198. An 8-year-old child with chronic renal failure is scheduled for an arteriovenous fistula. Laboratory studies include: Hb 6.5 g/dL, blood gas (on room air): PaO_2 97 mm Hg, $PaCO_2$ 29 mm Hg, pH 7.30, Na^+ 129 mEq/L, K^+ 5.5 mEq/L, Cl: 101 mEq/L, HCO_3: 15 mEq/L. Before inducing general anesthesia, which of the following abnormalities should be corrected?
    a. Anemia
    b. Metabolic acidosis
    c. Anemia, metabolic acidosis, and potassium concentration
    d. None of the above

199. A full term newborn is delivered by C section. 5 minutes after delivery, the baby has a heart rate of 110 bpm, is actively crying and coughing with good respiratory efforts and is vigorously moving all four extremities. The baby's SpO_2 is 70% on supplemental oxygen by face mask and has cyanosis of the face, trunk and extremities. What is this baby's 5-minute Apgar score?
    a. 6   b. 7
    c. 8   d. 9

200. MAC of inhalational anesthetics is the maximum at:
    a. Neonatal age   b. 1 – 3 years of age
    c. 6 – 12 months of age   d. 1 – 5 years of age

201. The following statements are *true* about gastroschisis, *except*:
    a. Covering sac is absent
    b. Associated systemic congenital anomalies are very common
    c. Maternal age < 20 years is a significant risk factor
    d. Herniation of contents occurs lateral to the umbilicus

202. The most common cause of OSA in children is:
    a. Obesity
    b. Adenotonsillar hypertrophy
    c. Craniofacial anomalies
    d. Hypotonia

203. The most common cause of anaphylaxis in a child undergoing surgery under anesthesia is due to:
    a. Muscle relaxants   b. Latex
    c. Antibiotics   d. Colloids

204. Under anesthesia, maximum heat loss in children occurs via:
    a. Conduction   b. Convection
    c. Radiation   d. Evaporation

205. Interruption of the aortic arch is most common in which syndrome:
    a. DiGeorge syndrome   b. Down's syndrome
    c. Turner syndrome   d. Alagille's syndrome

206. Local anesthetic having intrinsic vasoconstrictive activity is:
    a. Bupivacaine   b. Ropivacaine
    c. Levobupivacaine   d. Lignocaine

207. Normal PaO_2 in neonates is:
    a. 40–55 mm Hg   b. 55–70 mm Hg
    c. 70–85 mm Hg   d. 85–100 mm Hg

208. Blood volume in a premature infant is:
    a. 100–120 mL/kg
    b. 90–100 mL/kg
    c. 80 mL/kg
    d. 70 mL/kg

209. Regarding respiratory physiology in infants all are true, except:
    a. Airway is highly compliant
    b. Chestwall is highly compliant
    c. Diaphragm has predominantly type 1 muscle fibers
    d. Negative intrathoracic pressure is poorly maintained

210. The minimal standard for reprocessing laryngoscopes is:
    a. Sterilization
    b. High level disinfection
    c. Intermediate level disinfection
    d. Low level disinfection

211. All the following are tools for pain assessment, except:
    a. FLACC
    b. FACES scale
    c. PRISM score
    d. PIPP

212. Dubowitz scoring is a method:
    a. To evaluate airway in children
    b. To assess gestational age in infants
    c. To assess responsiveness in neonates
    d. To assess if the child is ready for discharge from PACU

213. Which statement is true about the concept of context-sensitive half-time of a drug?
    a. It helps determine the duration of action of a drug infusion after stopping the infusion
    b. It determines the time required for the drug to be eliminated
    c. It is not dependent on drug distribution
    d. It is a concept used to determine absorption by tissues

214. Which of the following contributes to the dead space in a circle system?
    a. CO_2 absorber
    b. Breathing reservoir bag
    c. Length of tubing from the unidirectional valve to the Y-piece
    d. Distance from the Y-piece to the terminal bronchioles

215. With regards to the ultrasound-guided TAP block which is true?
    a. The transversus abdominis plane is best visualized in the midline of the abdomen
    b. When advancing the needle during TAP blocks, the needle tip is best seen with an in plane needle view
    c. There is no need to visualize the spread of local anesthetic with this technique
    d. A "posterior" TAP block will spread to cover T7–T9 dermatomes only

216. Which one of the following statements regarding desflurane, is true?
    a. It boils at 25°C
    b. It is used safely in subjects with malignant hyperpyrexia
    c. It does not prolong the duration of action of muscle relaxants
    d. It is the least potent among the currently used agents

217. Regarding sevoflurane, which of the following is not true?
    a. Has a minimal alveolar concentration (MAC) of approximately 2%
    b. Has the lowest saturated vapor pressure among the currently used agents
    c. Is 2% metabolized by the liver
    d. Can cause hepatitis due to compound A formation

218. Which of the following vaporizers is not tilting proof?
    a. Aladin cassette vaporizer
    b. Maquet injector
    c. Drager DIVA
    d. TEC 7

219. In mechanical variable bypass vaporizers, metals are included in construction, as following, except:
    a. Heat sinks
    b. Conductors of electricity
    c. Conductors of heat
    d. Thermostats

220. When using agent gas monitoring, all of the following are measured in v/v%, except:
    a. FiO_2
    b. MAC
    c. Et agent
    d. $EtCO_2$

221. Which of the following cannot be delivered through a mechanical variable bypass vaporizer?
    a. Halothane
    b. Isoflurane
    c. Sevoflurane
    d. Desflurane

222. Which of the following vaporizers is classified as thermobuffered?
    a. TEC 5
    b. Dräger 2000
    c. Oxford miniature vaporizer
    d. Aladin cassette vaporizer

223. Which volatile agent is not an ether?
    a. Halothane
    b. Isoflurane
    c. Sevoflurane
    d. Desflurane

224. Which of the following has the lowest blood gas partition coefficient?

a. Desflurane
b. Nitrous oxide
c. Sevoflurane
d. Xenon

225. Which volatile agent is susceptible to degradation by Lewis acids?
    a. Desflurane
    b. Nitrous oxide
    c. Sevoflurane
    d. Xenon

226. Which of the following is a draw over vaporizer?
    a. Dräger 2000
    b. Oxford miniature vaporizer
    c. TEC 2
    d. Boyle's ether bottle

227. Which of the following can function as a bubble through vaporizer?
    a. Dual circuit gas vapor blender
    b. Aladin cassette vaporizer
    c. TEC 8 vaporizer
    d. Boyle's ether bottle

228. The filling systems used in modern vaporizers are primarily meant to:
    a. Prevent misfilling
    b. Prevent tipping
    c. Prevent pressurizing effect
    d. Prevent simultaneous use of two vaporizers

229. All of the following are vaporizer exclusion systems, *except*:
    a. Select-a-tec
    b. Dräger interlock I
    c. Dräger interlock II
    d. Keyed filling systems

230. All of the following are *true* regarding volatile anesthetic reflectors (AnaConDa and Mirus) used to deliver volatile anesthetics in ICU, *except*:
    a. It is an HME filter with a layer of activated charcoal
    b. The filter is intended for use for not more than 24 hours
    c. End tidal agent monitoring is not desirable
    d. Hemodynamic parameters should be monitored

231. Regarding the use of volatile anesthetic reflectors (AnaConDa and Mirus), in ICU, all of the following are *true, except*:
    a. Isoflurane, sevoflurane and desflurane can be delivered
    b. Could be used to treat refractory bronchospasm and status epilepticus
    c. The same filter can be used as long as the patient is ventilated
    d. Contains activated charcoal

232. Regarding variable bypass vaporizers, it is *true* that:
    a. Temperature compensation is not needed
    b. Performance is not significantly altered by changes in ambient pressure
    c. Splitting ratio depends on the blood gas solubility
    d. Wicks do not alter the extent of vaporization

233. Desflurane can be delivered via the Aladin cassette vaporizers and ADU systems because:
    a. Desflurane is highly volatile
    b. There is no loss of latent heat of vaporization
    c. This is an electronic variable bypass vaporizer
    d. Desflurane is the least potent (Mac 6%) of the volatile agents currently used

234. About the dual circuit gas vapor blenders, the following statement is *true*:
    a. It can be filled while in use
    b. Deliver the same output in partial pressure (mmHg), irrespective of ambient pressure
    c. Are designed to deliver desflurane, isoflurane and sevoflurane
    d. Have wicks

235. The safety features of mechanical variable bypass vaporizers include all of the following, *except*:
    a. Filling systems
    b. Vaporizer exclusion systems
    c. Audio visual alarms
    d. The Fraser Sweatman pin-index system

236. The safety features of electronic variable bypass vaporizers (Aladin cassette) include all of the following, *except*:
    a. Hypoxic guard
    b. Vaporizer exclusion systems
    c. Audio visual alarms – liquid levels
    d. The Fraser Sweatman pin-index system

237. Regarding modern injection vaporizers, all of the following are *true, except*:
    a. During the daily workstation pre-use check, vaporizers are automatically tested with respect to functionality and leaks
    b. Are tilting proof
    c. Vaporizer output is altered by changing the duration and speed of injection of the liquid agent
    d. Total fresh gas flow must increase to increase vaporizer output

238. Regarding dual circuit gas vapor blenders, all of the following features are *correct, except*:
    a. Electrically heated, thermostatically controlled
    b. Constant-temperature, pressurized
    c. Electromechanically coupled dual-circuit blenders
    d. Vaporizer in circuit location

239. All of the following are common sites of vaporizer leaks, *except*:
    a. Loose filler caps
    b. Vaporizer not seated properly

c. Missing O ring at port valve
d. Concentration control dial

240. **Which of the following vaporizers does not require electricity to function?**
    a. Mechanical variable bypass vaporizers
    b. Dual circuit gas vapor blenders
    c. Electronic variable bypass vaporizers
    d. Injection type vaporizers

241. **Complete the sentence with the most appropriate option: Risk of postoperative complications is significantly increased and short and long-term survival:**
    a. Is reduced with the transfusion of red cells that were <14 days old
    b. Is reduced with the transfusion of red cells that were >14 days old
    c. Is independent of the age of red cells transfused
    d. Is reduced only after 35 days of storage

242. **Blood transfusion has an immunomodulatory effect upon the recipient which may be associated with better outcomes after, all of these, *except*:**
    a. Renal transplantation
    b. Cardiac transplantation
    c. Liver transplantation
    d. Cancer recurrence

243. **Blood transfusion has an immunomodulatory effect upon the recipient which may be associated with worse outcomes after, all of these, *except*:**
    a. Perioperative infection
    b. Metastasis
    c. Liver transplantation
    d. Cancer recurrence

244. **Which of the following is diagnostic of transfusion-associated circulatory overload (TACO):**
    a. The chest X-ray shows interstitial edema, possibly in association with cardiomegaly
    b. A post-transfusion to pre-transfusion brain natriuretic peptide ratio of >1.5
    c. Acute respiratory distress, tachycardia, relative hypertension, raised central venous pressure
    d. Natriuretic pulmonary edema, and positive fluid balance

245. **Regarding FFP, the following is not *true*:**
    a. Fresh refers to timing from collection to freezing
    b. Frozen refers to the long-term storage condition
    c. FFP transfusion must be ABO compatible
    d. AB is the universal recipient type

246. **Regarding FFP, all the statements are *correct*, *except*:**
    a. Collected in citrate-containing anticoagulation solution
    b. Frozen within 8 hours of collection
    c. Stored at -30°C for up to 1 year
    d. Deficient in fibrinogen

247. **Regarding fresh frozen plasma, all of the following are *true*, *except*:**
    a. It contains all of the clotting factors
    b. It contains fibrinogen (400–900 mg/unit)
    c. It contains plasma proteins (particularly albumin)
    d. There are no added anticoagulants

248. **The indications for administration of FFP are, all of the following, *except*:**
    a. Prophylaxis if the coagulation tests are deranged
    b. Volume expansion
    c. Albumin deficiency
    d. Active bleeding and an International Normalized Ratio (INR) greater than 1.5

249. **Regarding the classification of blood groups, which of the following is not *true*?**
    a. It is based on the presence of different oligosaccharide antigens (agglutinogens) present on red cell membranes and agglutinins present in the plasma
    b. There are 29 agglutinogen-agglutinin systems
    c. Most hemolytic transfusion reactions involve the ABO and Rhesus (Rh) systems
    d. In the ABO system, Type AB individuals have circulating plasma anti-A and anti-B antibodies

250. **Due to repeated RBC transfusion in patients of hemosiderosis, all the following are *true*, *except*:**
    a. The body has no effective mechanism for excreting iron other than by blood loss
    b. Repeated transfusions can lead to iron accumulation with deposition in the liver, heart, pancreas, and endocrine organs
    c. This does not ultimately lead to cirrhosis, cardiomyopathy, diabetes, arthritis, and testicular failure
    d. The onset of iron overload, may be delayed or offset by the use of recurrent venesection or iron chelating agents like deferasirox

251. **Regarding transfusion-related bacterial contamination all of the following are *true*, *except*:**
    a. The major bacterial contaminants are skin organisms acquired at the time of donation.
    b. Discarding the initial flow of blood before it enters the collection bag has been highly effective in reducing bacterial contamination
    c. Platelets have the highest risk of bacterial contamination (1:2000) because they are stored at room temperature
    d. The risk with red cell concentrates is the highest

252. Regarding *incorrect* blood component transfusions, which of the following is untrue?
    a. More common with increasing age
    b. More common with decreasing age
    c. Predominantly attributable to the failure of effective identity checks before transfusion
    d. Anesthetized patients are at high risk as they are unable to confirm their details and access to identity bracelets can be difficult in theatre

253. Regarding viral contamination of blood, it is untrue that:
    a. Leucodepletion has no effect on viral transmission
    b. It is now extremely rare due to the suspension of red cells in minimal amounts of plasma
    c. Donated blood is routinely screened for human immunodeficiency virus (HIV), hepatitis B and C, and human T cell lymphoma virus 1
    d. Leucodepletion has greatly reduced the transmission of cytomegalovirus (CMV)

254. All of the following changes are expected in stored blood, *except:*
    a. Decrease in clotting factors
    b. Acidic pH
    c. Decrease in potassium
    d. Decrease in 2,3 DPG

255. The risk of which transfusion transmitted infection is highest?
    a. Viral
    b. Bacterial
    c. Protozoal
    d. All of the above carry similar risk

256. The risk of bacterial contamination is greatest when the patient is transfused with:
    a. Fresh frozen plasma
    b. Platelets
    c. Whole blood
    d. Packed cells

257. Regarding bacterial contamination of platelets, all of the following are *true, except:*
    a. The most common contaminants are gram positive bacteria
    b. Contamination is most likely to occur during donor phlebotomy
    c. A small inoculum can proliferate due to storage at room temperature
    d. Pooled platelet concentrates from buffy coats have a lower bacterial contamination rate compared to apheresis platelets

258. Regarding the COVID-19 epidemic and transfusion of blood products, all of the following are *true, except:*
    a. No cases of transfusion-transmission were ever reported for the other two coronaviruses that emerged during the past two decades (SARS, MERS-CoV)
    b. Respiratory viruses are generally not known to be transmitted by donation or transfusion
    c. Individuals are not at risk of contracting COVID-19 through the blood donation process or via a blood transfusion
    d. Asymptomatic individuals with past history of COVID infection should be barred from blood donation

259. Regarding the COVID-19 epidemic and blood donation, all of the following are *true, except:*
    a. Individuals who received a COVID-19 vaccine cannot donate blood
    b. Individuals who received a nonreplicating, inactivated, or mRNA-based COVID-19 vaccine can donate blood without a waiting period
    c. Individuals who received a live-attenuated viral COVID-19 vaccine, refrain from donating blood for a short waiting period (e.g., 14 days) after receipt of the vaccine
    d. Individuals who are uncertain about which COVID-19 vaccine was administered, refrain from donating for a short waiting period (e.g., 14 days) if it is possible that the individual received a live-attenuated viral vaccine

260. Regarding the COVID-19 epidemic and blood donation, all of the following are *true, except:*
    a. FDA does not recommend using COVID-19 laboratory tests to screen routine blood donors
    b. The blood establishment's responsible physician must evaluate prospective donors and determine eligibility
    c. Individuals diagnosed with COVID-19 or who are suspected of having COVID-19, and who had symptomatic disease, need not refrain from donating blood
    d. The donor must be in good health and meet all donor eligibility criteria on the day of donation

261. In which congenital cardiac defect, intravenous induction of anesthesia is fastest?
    a. Atrial septal defect
    b. Ventricular septal defect
    c. Congenital aortic stenosis
    d. Tetralogy of Fallot

262. Male child of 6 years underwent right inguinal hernia repair under general anesthesia with ilioinguinal and iliohypogastric block. Postoperatively he can not extend his right leg at knee. What is your diagnosis?
    a. Spread of local anesthetic to the femoral nerve
    b. Nerve injury due to surgical positioning

c. Epidural spread of local anesthetic
d. Direct injury to the ilioinguinal nerve

263. **Which property of surfactant is responsible in preventing alveolar collapse?**
    a. Increases alveolar diffusion
    b. Decreases lung compliance
    c. Decreases alveolar surface tension
    d. Decreases transpulmonary pressure

264. **What would be the best plan of airway management in a 3-year-old child with intestinal obstruction coming for emergency exploratory laparotomy?**
    a. Classic rapid sequence induction and intubation with uncuffed ETT
    b. Controlled rapid sequence induction and intubation with cuffed ETT
    c. Classic rapid sequence induction and intubation with cuffed ETT
    d. Controlled rapid sequence induction and intubation with uncuffed ETT

265. **Which of the following is the *correct* statement about cleft lip and palate?**
    a. It is the commonest congenital abnormality
    b. Cleft palate cannot occur without cleft lip
    c. It is more common in males and more often found on the left side
    d. Associated abnormalities are very rare

266. **Which of the following is not *correct* about airway obstruction after cleft palate repair?**
    a. Is most likely to occur in children with preoperative airway problems
    b. May be treated with insertion of a nasopharyngeal airway
    c. Oropharyngeal airways should be avoided
    d. Will always require re-intubation

267. **What may not increase the risk of perioperative respiratory adverse events (prae) in children with urti?**
    a. Urti > 4 weeks ago
    b. Use of supraglottic airway device or endotracheal tube
    c. Preexisting pulmonary disorder
    d. Airway surgery

268. **Delayed recovery from anesthesia in premature and ex-premature infants is not due to:**
    a. Hypoglycemia / hypothermia / acidosis
    b. Broncho-pulmonary dysplasia
    c. Immature liver and kidney functions
    d. Intracranial bleed

269. **Congenital hypertrophic pyloric stenosis (CHPS) is associated with:**
    a. Hyperkalemia
    b. Hyperchloremia
    c. Metabolic acidosis
    d. Metabolic alkalosis

270. **A 12 year boy is brought to emergency with testicular torsion. Child is NBM for solids for 6 hours. Surgeon wants to operate immediately. What would be your response?**
    a. Take him to the or, consider it emergent, rapid-sequence induction and intubation (rsii)
    b. Wait for 2 more hours, consider it urgent, rsii
    c. He is adequately fasting, elective, intubation
    d. Wait for 2 hours, elective, intubation

271. **The first sign of accidental intrathecal la injection following the placement of caudal. Epidural in a 1-year-old spontaneously breathing infant with laryngeal mask:**
    a. Hypotension
    b. Bradycardia
    c. Desaturation and apnea
    d. Tachycardia

272. **For MRI under sedation in pediatric patients, what is essential to prevent burns injury?**
    a. Screening the patient for metal implants in zone IV
    b. Using MR-safe monitors
    c. Curling the monitor cable on top of the patient's hand
    d. Cooling the patient during the MRI scan

273. **Which of the following child is at the highest risk for developing postoperative nausea and vomiting (PONV)?**
    a. 1 Year infant undergoing circumcision under inhalational anesthesia
    b. 15 Years female undergoing squint surgery with h/o motion sickness
    c. 5 years female undergoing close reduction of distal radius fracture under tiva
    d. 17 years male, with h/o smoking, undergoing cystoscopy under total intravenous anesthesia

274. **Pediatric airway has:**
    a. More caudal position of larynx as compared to adult
    b. Less acute angulation of epiglottis
    c. Glottic opening as the narrowest part of airway, with elliptical cross-section
    d. Longer trachea as compared to adults

275. **Anesthetic management of a 6-year-old with down syndrome includes all of the following, *except*:**
    a. Continue anticonvulsant medications
    b. Heavy sedation since these kids are aggressive
    c. Prepare for manual in line neck stabilization
    d. X-ray neck should be reviewed to rule out atlantooccipital instability

276. **Positive-pressure ventilation with a face mask is contraindicated in:**
    a. Laryngospasm
    b. Congenital diaphragmatic hernia
    c. Apnea
    d. Asthma

277. **The total dose of midazolam that may be given orally as premedication is:**
    a. 0.2 mg/kg, ≤10 mg
    b. 0.3 mg/kg, ≤15 mg
    c. 0.75 mg/kg, ≤25 mg
    d. 0.5 mg/kg, ≤20 mg

278. **To protect lungs in a child with tracheoesophageal fistula, this is not indicated:**
    a. Nil by mouth
    b. Upright position
    c. Intermittent suction of upper blind esophageal pouch
    d. Prophylactic intravenous steroids

279. **Basic metabolic rate and oxygen requirement in children is:**
    a. Least till 2 years of age
    b. Same as adults
    c. Highest till 2 years of age
    d. Decreases after puberty

280. **Most reliable sign of accidental IV injection of LA containing 1:200000 adrenaline in children is:**
    a. Tachycardia
    b. ST segment, T wave amplitude changes
    c. Bradycardia
    d. Hypertension

281. **One of the best predictors of difficult airway in the morbidly obese is:**
    a. Mallampati score > 3
    b. Neck circumference > 42 cm
    c. BMI > 50 kg/m^2
    d. The presence of a beard

282. **Advantages of ramped position for induction of anesthesia in morbidly obese include all except:**
    a. Reduced dyspnea and increased comfort for the patient
    b. Functional residual capacity is maintained
    c. Bag-mask ventilation and laryngoscopy is facilitated
    d. Laryngoscopic response is reduced

283. **Standard technique for intraoperative thromboprophylaxis in morbidly obese is:**
    a. Intermittent pneumatic calf compression
    b. Graduated compression stockinets
    c. Low molecular weight heparin
    d. Temporary IVC filter

284. **Essential monitoring for bariatric anesthesia includes:**
    a. Depth of anesthesia monitoring and neuromuscular block monitoring
    b. Invasive blood pressure monitoring
    c. Central venous pressure monitoring
    d. Transesophageal echocardiography

285. **Which of the following statements is *true* regarding drug usage for bariatric anesthesia?**
    a. Long acting opioids and sedatives are safe if anesthesia depth is monitored
    b. Dosing should be based upon lean body weight and titrated to effect
    c. Sevoflurane is preferred over desflurane
    d. No need to reverse non-depolarizing muscle relaxant if one is monitoring the block

286. **OS-MRS, obesity-surgery mortality risk score used for risk prediction does not include:**
    a. BMI > 50 kg/m^2
    b. Hypertensive male > 45 years of age
    c. Risk factors for PE (previous VTE, preoperative vena cava filter, OSA/OHS, right heart failure, pulmonary hypertension)
    d. Good preoperative optimization of comorbidities and compliance

287. **Postoperative HDU/ICU care is usually not required for gastric bypass surgery for obesity if patient has:**
    a. Untreated pre-existing comorbidities
    b. Indicated high risk (OS-MRS score 4–5 or METS <4)
    c. Open abdominal surgical procedure
    d. Treated and optimized obstructive sleep apnea

288. **This practice may not be useful to increase safe apnea duration in obese patient before intubation:**
    a. Preoxygenation with 100% oxygen for 5 minutes or till end-expiratory oxygen (FeO$_2$) concentration > 90%
    b. Bag-mask ventilation with PEEP before endotracheal intubation
    c. Application of CPAP in 25° head high position
    d. Apneic oxygenation

289. **Which obese patient of the following could be appropriate for day case surgery?**
    a. OS-MRS (obesity surgery–mortality risk score) 4–5
    b. Unstable cardiorespiratory system
    c. METs < 4
    d. METs > 4, OSA/OHS effectively treated by NIV and able to continue VTE prophylaxis at home if required

290. **This obese patient can not be discharged from PACU after surgery:**
    a. Stable hemodynamics with minimal oxygen requirement

b. Evidence of hypoventilation and desaturation if not stimulated
c. Wide awake in sitting position with CPAP initiated in PACU
d. Surgery done under regional anesthesia, patient pain free

291. What would be the predicted postoperative FEV_1 of a patient who is posted for left lower lobectomy and has a preoperative FEV_1 of 70%?
a. 59%
b. 43%
c. 53%
d. 38%

292. Apart from ventilation what is the other function of the ECOM double lumen tube?
a. Temperature monitoring
b. Cardiac output monitoring
c. Anesthesia gas monitoring
d. Extravascular lung water measurement

293. In which part of the GI tract is vitamin B12 absorbed?
a. Ileum
b. Duodenum
c. Antrum of stomach
d. Jejunum

294. Which cells are known as pacemaker cells of GI tract?
a. Chief cells
b. Paneth cells
c. Interstitial cells of Cajal
d. Parietal cells

295. Which of the following situations will be most likely associated with delayed gastric emptying?
a. Patient taking oral erythromycin
b. Patient on a high dose of noradrenaline
c. Patient receiving epidural analgesia containing bupivacaine in postoperative period
d. Patient receiving metoclopramide for nausea

296. ENIGMA-2 trial evaluated:
a. Effect of nitrous oxide on perioperative cardiovascular events and mortality in patients undergoing major non-cardiac surgery
b. Effect of opioids on perioperative cardiovascular events and mortality in patients undergoing non cardiac surgery
c. Effect of volatile anesthetics and total intravenous anesthesia on perioperative cardiovascular events and mortality in patients undergoing major non cardiac surgery
d. Effect of epidural analgesia on perioperative cardiovascular events and mortality in patients undergoing major non-cardiac surgery

297. Which of the following organs is not supplied by coeliac plexus?
a. Ileum
b. Adrenal glands
c. Spleen
d. Uterus

298. Which of the following neuropeptides causes vasodilatation?
a. Vasoactive intestinal polypeptide
b. Neuropeptide Y
c. Neuropeptide U
d. Endothelin-1

299. Which of the following is not a characteristic feature of 'mass reflex' which is seen in spinal cord injury?
a. Dramatic fall in BP
b. Dramatic rise in BP
c. Flushing of the skin above the level of injury
d. Headache

300. Which of the following causes of hypoxemia does not respond to increase in FiO_2?
a. V/Q mismatch
b. Diffusion impairment
c. Shunt
d. Hypoventilation

301. In which zone of lung, alveolar pressure can exceed pulmonary arterial and venous pressure during positive pressure ventilation?
a. Zone 1
b. Zone 2
c. Zone 3
d. Zone 4

302. Which of the following conditions is least likely associated with shunt?
a. Atelectasis
b. Consolidation
c. Pulmonary edema
d. Emphysema

303. According to Laplace's law, the left ventricular wall stress is maintained constant in aortic stenosis by:
a. Increasing LV radius
b. Increasing LV thickness
c. Increasing the heart rate
d. Increasing the end diastolic ventricular volume

304. What is the maximum dose of 20% lipid emulsion dose while treating local anesthetic systemic toxicity?
a. 5 mL/kg
b. 20 mL/kg
c. 12 mL/kg
d. 6 mL/kg

305. Which of the following volumes can not be measured by direct spirometry?
    a. Inspiratory reserve volume
    b. Expiratory reserve volume
    c. Vital capacity
    d. Residual volume

306. How much is the contribution of the glycocalyx to the intravascular volume?
    a. 0.1%
    b. 2%
    c. 10%
    d. 40%

307. Which statement regarding dantrolene is *true*?
    a. The initial dose of dantrolene in malignant hyperthermia is 8 mg/kg
    b. Dantrolene should be reconstituted in normal saline
    c. Dantrolene has a half-life of 10 hours
    d. Dantrolene is a drug of choice for treatment of myasthenia gravis

308. According to 2018 ASRA guidelines for regional anesthesia in patients receiving anticoagulant therapy, how long rivaroxaban should be discontinued prior to performing a neuraxial block?
    a. 24 hours
    b. 48 hours
    c. 60 hours
    d. 72 hours

309. Which of the following statement is *true* regarding NAP 5 (national audit project)?
    a. The overall estimated incidence of AAGA (accidental awareness during general anesthesia) was found to be 1:1000.
    b. Majority of AAGA events occurred in the maintenance phase of anesthesia.
    c. ASA physical status was not found as a risk factor for AAGA
    d. Incidence was higher when neuromuscular blockade was not used.

310. Bainbridge reflex is:
    a. Tachycardia due to ventricular irritation due to noxious stimuli
    b. Triad of bradycardia, hypotension and coronary artery dilatation due to stimulation of LV wall mechanoceptors
    c. Bradycardia and decreased myocardial contractility in response to hypoxia
    d. Tachycardia in response to increased right atrial filling pressures

311. The dose of adrenaline for pulseless cardiac arrest in children is:
    a. 0.05 mg/kg
    b. 0.04 mg/kg
    c. 0.02 mg/kg
    d. 0.01 mg/kg

312. Which statement regarding EEG is *true*?
    a. The normal EEG pattern in awake patient is in the delta frequency range
    b. Deep sleep and anesthesia generally exhibit beta frequency signals on EEG
    c. EEG is a summation of excitatory and inhibitory presynaptic potentials produced in cortical gray matter
    d. For a reliable isoelectric EEG, the interelectrode impedances should be less than 10,000 ohms but more than 100 ohms

313. Which one of following is *true* regarding ARDS?
    a. The goal of mechanical ventilation is to maintain normal PO_2 and PCO_2
    b. A normal PCWP indicative of noncardiogenic pulmonary edema is required for ARDS diagnosis
    c. Adding PEEP during mechanical ventilation decreases the cyclical shear stress injury
    d. "Baby lung" concept of ARDS is amount of non-aerated lung in ARDS is roughly equivalent to the lung tissue of 6-year-old boy

314. The term "coroner's clot" is used for:
    a. Blood clot in the coronary circulation
    b. Blood clot in cerebral vasculature
    c. Total airway obstruction and death after tracheal extubation due to blood clot following nasal surgery
    d. Pulmonary embolism

315. Which statement is *true* regarding the anesthesia for laser surgery?
    a. Addition of nitrous oxide reduces the oxygen concentration and thereby reduces the risk of airway fires during laser surgery
    b. Laser shield II tube is made up of PVC and is wrapped by a coated aluminium tape
    c. The laser flex tube has a unique self-inflating foam sponge-filled cuff
    d. Merocel laser guard has been FDA approved to wrap the endotracheal tubes during laser surgery

316. Choose the *correct* option regarding CO_2 absorbers:
    a. Barium hydroxide is the main component of baralyme
    b. Sevoflurane causes greatest production of carbon monoxide upon reacting with the CO_2 absorber
    c. Unlike soda lime, lithium hydroxide-based absorbers do not need an additional catalyst
    d. Absorptive capacity of soda lime is more than lithium hydroxide containing CO_2 absorbers

317. Which of the following LMA is MRI compatible?
    a. LMA Supreme
    b. LMA Classic
    c. LMA Proseal
    d. i-gel

318. A 65-year-old gentleman is undergoing open gastrectomy surgery. Patient has a oropharyngeal temperature reading of 34.5°C. What is the most important mechanism of heat loss for this patient?
    a. Conduction
    b. Convection
    c. Evaporation
    d. Radiation

319. What is "open lung" concept?
    a. Using recruitment methods and PEEP to open the collapsed alveolar units
    b. Using spontaneous ventilation to avoid atelectasis and alveolar collapse
    c. Applying CPAP to non-ventilated lung during one lung ventilation
    d. Using prone position for ventilation to avoid atelectrauma

320. Which statement is not *true* regarding driving pressure?
    a. It is calculated as peak airway pressure minus PEEP in patients who are mechanically ventilated without any spontaneous efforts
    b. It is the ratio of tidal volume (Vt) to static compliance of respiratory system (Crs)
    c. If increasing the PEEP causes decrease in the driving pressure; it indicates increase in lung compliance
    d. Higher driving pressures are associated with higher mortality

321. Which definition is used to define ARDS?
    a. Gurd definition
    b. Berlin definition
    c. Jone criteria
    d. Wilson score

322. In Schonfeld fat embolism syndrome index, maximum score is given to which sign/symptom?
    a. Petechial rash
    b. Diffuse alveolar infiltrates
    c. Tachycardia
    d. Hypoxemia (PaO$_2$ < 70 with FiO$_2$ 100%)

323. In auscultatory method for BP measurement described by Korotkoff, the diastolic BP is measured in which phase?
    a. Phase I
    b. Phase II
    c. Phase III
    d. Phase IV or V

324. Which of the following techniques for BP measurement is the 'Riva-Rocci' method?
    a. Auscultatory method
    b. Noninvasive BP by oscillometry
    c. Disappearance of radial pulse by palpation during cuff inflation
    d. Invasive BP monitoring

325. Compared to central aortic pressure waveform, the dorsalis pedis arterial waveform will have:
    a. Higher systolic and higher diastolic pressure
    b. Lower systolic and lower diastolic pressure
    c. Lower systolic and higher diastolic pressure
    d. Higher systolic and lower diastolic pressure

326. Pulsus paradoxus is:
    a. Exaggerated inspiratory fall in systolic arterial pressure during quiet breathing
    b. Exaggerated inspiratory fall in systolic arterial pressure during deep breathing
    c. Exaggerated inspiratory fall in diastolic arterial pressure during quiet breathing
    d. Exaggerated expiratory rise in systolic arterial pressure during quiet breathing

327. Which of the following condition will have Pulses alternans?
    a. Atrial fibrillation
    b. Severe ventricular systolic dysfunction
    c. Trivial aortic regurgitation
    d. Mild mitral stenosis

328. Which of the following is NOT a feature of SIADH?
    a. Urinary sodium levels are generally <20 mEq/L
    b. Patients with mild to moderate symptoms can be treated with restriction of fluid intake
    c. SIADH patients are unable to excrete dilute urine even after water loading.
    d. Patients have hypertonic urine relative to plasma

329. Which of the following statement is *correct* regarding the neuromuscular junction:
    a. The synaptic cleft is 2 nanometres wide
    b. The depths of the folds are densely populated with acetylcholine receptors
    c. Nerve fibers converge on the motor end-plate of the muscle fiber
    d. The terminal portion of the motor neurone is unmyelinated

330. Which of the following statements regarding the ligaments of the vertebral column is *correct*?
    a. The anterior longitudinal ligament is found around the anterior aspect of the vertebral foramen
    b. The ligamentum flavum connects the adjacent laminae
    c. The interspinous ligaments are continuous from the cervical vertebrae to lumbar vertebrae
    d. The supraspinous ligament provide much of natural recoil of the natural recoil of the spine and become thicker in the lower regions of the spine

331. Which statement regarding thirst is *incorrect*?
    a. The thirst center is sensitive to angiotensin II
    b. The osmoreceptors that sense osmolality of body fluids are located in posterior hypothalamus
    c. The thirst center has osmoreceptors that are sensitive to extracellular tonicity
    d. Satiety from thirst is induced by activation of pharyngeal receptors sensitive to water consumption

332. Which of the following statement is *false* regarding the circle of Willis
    a. Posterior cerebral artery is a branch of the internal carotid artery
    b. Internal carotid artery gives off ophthalmic artery
    c. Posterior communicating arteries connects the internal carotid arteries to the posterior cerebral arteries
    d. Anterior communicating artery connects the two anterior cerebral arteries

333. Muscle responsible for opening mouth is:
    a. Masseter
    b. Medial pterygoid
    c. Lateral pterygoid
    d. Temporalis

334. Muscles responsible for protrusion if chin are all except:
    a. Lateral pterygoid
    b. Suprahyoid
    c. Masseter
    d. Medial pterygoid

335. Which of the following is not a temporomandibular joint ligament?
    a. Stylomandibular
    b. Temporomandibular
    c. Tympanomandibular
    d. Sphenomandibular

336. Which of the following is *true* about the curvatures of the vertebral column:
    a. Primary curves are concave forward
    b. Lumbar curve is a primary curvature
    c. Thoracic curve develops when infant starts walking
    d. Lumbar lordosis appears when the infant starts supporting its head

337. A man presents with complaints of chest pain. On examination it is found that there is pericarditis with pericardial effusion. The pain is mediated by:
    a. Deep cardiac plexus
    b. Superficial cardiac plexus
    c. Phrenic nerve
    d. Subcostal nerve

338. Which of the following is *incorrect* regarding the role and location of central chemoreceptors in the control of breathing?
    a. The central chemoreceptors are located near the dorsal surface of the pons
    b. Central chemoreceptors respond rapidly to changes in carbon dioxide tension in the blood
    c. The pH of cerebrospinal fluid is slightly acidic compared with plasma
    d. Respiratory acidosis causes a greater increase in ventilation than metabolic acidosis

339. Which of the following statements about the intercostal nerves is *incorrect*?
    a. The intercostal nerves contain sensory, motor and autonomic fibers
    b. The intercostal nerves run between the internal intercostal muscle and the transversus thoracic muscle
    c. The anterior rami of nerves T1–T11 form the intercostal nerves
    d. A chest drain should be inserted at the inferior aspect of the intercostal space

340. Which of the following statement regarding the cranial vault in a healthy adult is *true*:
    a. The mass of a human brain is approximately 1000 g
    b. 85% of the cranial volume is occupied by brain parenchyma
    c. Total volume of cerebrospinal fluid in the cranial vault is 150 mL
    d. Early compensation for raised intracranial pressure (ICP) includes reduced production of cerebrospinal fluid

341. Which of the following statements regarding the internal jugular vein is not *true*?
    a. The internal jugular vein drains the sigmoid sinus
    b. The internal jugular vein begins at the foramen lacerum at the base of the skull
    c. Horner's syndrome is a recognized complication of attempted cannulation of the internal jugular vein
    d. The internal jugular vein contains a bicuspid valve near its termination

342. All of the following statements are *true* regarding the structural organization of a peripheral nerve fiber except:
    a. Blood–nerve barrier is formed by the endoneurium
    b. Individual nerve fiber is covered by endoneurium
    c. Each nerve fascicle is wrapped by perineurium
    d. Epineurium covers the entire nerve

343. Which of the following statements regarding peripheral nerves holds *true*?
    a. C-fibers carry proprioception and muscle tone

b. B-fibers are postganglionic axons of the autonomic nervous system
c. Conduction velocity of Aα fibers is 70–120 m/second
d. Thickness of C-fibers is 5–12 µm

344. Identify the *incorrect* statement regarding the anatomy of sacral canal:
   a. Sacral hiatus is roofed by the sacrococcygeal ligament
   b. Sacral hiatus is formed by inferior articular process of S5
   c. Sacrococcygeal ligament is an extension of ligamentum flavum
   d. The sacral canal contains cauda equina, spinal meninges, epidural venous plexus and adipose tissue

345. Which of the following statement is *False* with regards to celiac plexus?
   a. The celiac plexus is composed of pre- and postganglionic sympathetic, parasympathetic and visceral sensory afferents fibers
   b. The right celiac ganglion is slightly lower than the left ganglion
   c. Celiac plexus is the largest plexus of sympathetic nervous system that innervates the upper abdominal organs
   d. Celiac plexus block is also known as solar plexus block

346. Which of the following is not an anterior mediastinal mass?
   a. Teratoma
   b. Lymphoma
   c. Thymoma
   d. Bronchogenic cyst

347. *False* statement about right coronary artery (RCA) is:
   a. Diameter less than left coronary artery
   b. RCA arises from the anterior aortic sinus
   c. RCA supplies major part of right atrium and right ventricle
   d. RCA supplies to the right bundle branch

348. Coronary dominance is determined by:
   a. Posterior interventricular artery
   b. Anterior interventricular artery
   c. Circumflex artery
   d. Right coronary artery

349. Majority of oxygen consumption of the day in healthy adult results from:
   a. Electrical activity
   b. Volume work
   c. Pressure work
   d. Basal requirement

350. General sensation to the posterior one-third of the tongue is mediated by the:
   a. Hypoglossal nerve
   b. Vagus nerve
   c. Glossopharyngeal nerve
   d. Lingual nerve

351. Adult larynx extends from cervical spine level:
   a. C3–C4
   b. C3–C6
   c. C3–C5
   d. C4–C6

352. Which of the following statement is *incorrect*?
   a. Beyond the tertiary segmental bronchi, there are 20–25 generations of branching conducting bronchioles that eventually end as terminal bronchioles
   b. Due to the presence of the alveoli, the respiratory bronchioles are involved both in air transportation and gas exchange
   c. Each respiratory bronchiole gives rise to 2–11 alveolar ducts, each of which gives rise to 5–6 alveolar sacs
   d. New alveoli continue to develop until 2 years of age

353. Which of the following statement is not *true* regarding the relations of the right atrium?
   a. The SVC opens into the superior part of the right atrium at the level of the right 3rd costal cartilage
   b. The IVC opens into the inferior part of the right atrium almost in line with the SVC at the level of 5th costal cartilage
   c. The opening of the coronary sinus lies between the IVC orifice and the SVC orifice
   d. The interatrial septum has an oval, thumbprint-size depression, the oval fossa

354. In a heart with right-dominant coronary circulation which coronary artery supplies the AV bundle of the heart?
   a. Both the right and the left bundle branch of the AV bundle are supplied by the right coronary artery
   b. The right bundle of the AV bundle is supplied by the right coronary artery, the left bundle of the AV bundle is supplied by the left anterior descending artery
   c. Both the right and the left bundle branch of the AV bundle are supplied by the left coronary artery
   d. The right bundle of the AV bundle is supplied by the right coronary artery, the left bundle of the AV bundle is supplied by the left coronary artery

355. Regarding the anatomy of the mediastinum which of the following statement is *true*:
   a. The thymus lies in the posterior mediastinum

b. Lymphatics and lymph nodes are present only in the posterior mediastinum.
c. Posterior mediastinum contains the thoracic aorta, thoracic duct and lymphatic trunks
d. Posterior boundary of posterior mediastinum corresponds to T1–T4 vertebrae

356. Which of the following is not a content of posterior mediastinum?
    a. Descending thoracic aorta
    b. Thoracic duct
    c. Phrenic nerves
    d. Azygous vein

357. Lymph from the lower half of the body drains into:
    a. Cisterna chyli
    b. Right lymphatic duct
    c. Right brachiocephalic vein
    d. Pulmonary trunk

358. The esophageal opening in the diaphragm transmits:
    a. Azygous vein
    b. Vagus nerve
    c. Right phrenic nerve
    d. Thoracic duct

359. Which of the following muscles contributes in quiet respiration?
    a. External intercostal muscle
    b. Abdominal muscle
    c. None
    d. Internal intercostal muscle

360. Which statement about dead space is not *true*?
    a. Anatomical dead space is around 150 mL
    b. Total dead space is alveolar dead space + anatomical dead space
    c. In pulmonary embolism anatomical dead space increases
    d. Anatomical dead space remains constant

361. A 40-year-old female with TMJ ankylosis is scheduled for gap arthroplasty. Due to concern of challenging laryngoscopy, anesthesiologist plans awake fiberoptic intubation. In order to anesthetize posterior third of tongue, which nerve should be blocked?
    a. Cranial nerve V
    b. CN VII
    c. CN IX
    d. CN XII

362. All statements are *true* about cervical plexus *except*:
    a. It is formed by anterior division of C1–C4
    b. It lies superficial to sternocleidomastoid
    c. Tragus is supplied by auriculotemporal nerve
    d. It has sensory and motor branches

363. Uterine blood flow in non-pregnant adult female is approximately:
    a. 50 mL/min
    b. 100 mL/min
    c. 200 mL/min
    d. 500 mL/min

364. Uterine blood flow at term is:
    a. 5% of cardiac output
    b. 10% of cardiac output
    c. 20% of cardiac output
    d. 25% of cardiac output

365. Which of the following statement is *False* regarding the caval opening of diaphragm?
    a. The caval opening is an aperture in the central tendon
    b. Inferior vena cava and terminal branches of the right phrenic nerve pass through it
    c. It is the most inferior of the three large diaphragmatic apertures
    d. It widens during inspiration, and therefore the IVC during inspiration

366. The sympathetic part of the autonomic innervation of the abdominal viscera consists of the following, *except*:
    a. Lower thoracic splanchnic nerves
    b. Prevertebral sympathetic ganglia
    c. Abdominal aortic plexus and its extensions, the peri-arterial plexuses
    d. Pelvic splanchnic nerves

367. Which of the following statement is *true* regarding blood supply to the heart?
    a. Artery to SA node is more commonly a branch of left coronary artery
    b. "Left dominance" pattern is seen in almost 40% of hearts
    c. Right coronary artery originates from the posterior aortic sinus
    d. Dominance of the coronary arterial system depends on which artery gives rise to the posterior descending artery

368. Which of the following statement is *incorrect* regarding the deep cardiac plexus:
    a. It lies in front of tracheal bifurcation
    b. Receives branches from the cervical and upper four thoracic ganglia as well as the vagal branches
    c. The deep part of the cardiac plexus is larger
    d. The cardiac plexus is formed by sympathetic fibers alone

369. Which of the following statement is *true* about the thoracic duct:
    a. It enters the right side of the superior mediastinum
    b. It drains both upper limbs

c. It does not drain the right arm
d. It terminates in the inferior vena cava

370. All of the following parts of conducting system of the heart are supplied by right coronary artery, except:
a. SA node
b. AV node
c. AV bundle
d. Right bundle branch

371. Length of trachea in adults is:
a. 10–12 cm
b. 14–16 cm
c. 6–10 cm
d. None of above

372. Trachea bifurcates at the level of which vertebrae?
a. T2
b. T3
c. T4
d. T6

373. Normal area of mitral valve is:
a. 2–4 cm^2
b. 4–6 cm^2
c. 6–8 cm^2
d. 8–10 cm^2

374. Recommended tidal volume during one lung ventilation is:
a. 4–6 mL/kg actual body weight
b. 7–8 mL/kg ideal body weight
c. 4–6 mL/kg ideal body weight
d. 3 mL/kg actual body weight

375. The commonest indication for intraoperative use of lung separation techniques is:
a. Bronchopleural fistula
b. To facilitate surgical exposure
c. Lung hemorrhage
d. To improve gas exchange during lung resection surgery

376. Regarding lung isolation, a left sided double lumen tube should preferably be avoided in all of the following, except:
a. Left mainstem bronchus tumor
b. Left bronchotomy
c. Left lower lobectomy
d. Left pneumonectomy

377. Regarding hypoxic pulmonary vasoconstriction (HPV) during one lung ventilation, which of the following is true?
a. Vasodilators improve HPV
b. Inhalational agents should not be used during one lung ventilation
c. PEEP has no effect on HPV
d. HPV is primarily responsible for reducing shunt during OLV

378. Regarding flail segment of chest wall, the correct statement is:
a. Positive pressure ventilation is better than normal spontaneous breathing
b. Posterolateral thoracotomy is most common cause of flail segment
c. Chest drain is beneficial in management of flail chest
d. Epidural analgesia is mandatory for management of a flail chest

379. Which bronchial blocker has a bifurcated end with 2 bronchial cuffs?
a. Coopdech blocker
b. Arndt blocker
c. EZ blocker
d. Fuji Blocker

380. Regarding intercostal drain (chest drain), the correct statement is:
a. Negative pressure (suction) is commonly applied in the post pneumonectomy cavity
b. 2 chest drains viz. apical and basal are mandatory after lung resection surgery
c. Heimlich valve can be used in place of an underwater seal
d. 2 bottle system is inferior to one bottle system when large amount of liquid is to be drained

381. Regarding pulmonary function tests, the incorrect statement is:
a. Clinical practice guidelines for lung resection surgery commonly use the predicted postoperative forced vital capacity (PPO FVC) value to determine risk
b. The largest FVC and the largest FEV1 observed from all of the acceptable values are used for FEV1/FVC, even though the largest FVC and the largest FEV1 may not necessarily come from the same maneuver
c. The 2019 American Thoracic Society Update on standardization of spirometry requires 3 tests with FVC within 150 mL of each other for best validity of the test in adult patients
d. Diffusion capacity of lung for carbon monoxide is affected by the blood hemoglobin level

382. Regarding pulmonary function tests, the incorrect statement is:
a. DLCO is a more sensitive indicator of gas exchange abnormalities than arterial blood gas analysis
b. Flow volume loops are useful in differentiating between intrathoracic and extrathoracic variable obstruction
c. FEV1 may be low in both obstructive as well as restrictive lung conditions
d. Total lung capacity is the most important value for the interpretation of a standard spirometry test

383. On bronchoscopy, a clover leaf view (3 orifices) is seen in which structure?
a. Right main bronchus
b. Right upper lobe bronchus

c. Left main bronchus
d. Left upper lobe bronchus

384. Regarding flow of fluids, which statement is *false*?
   a. Hagen Poiseuilles equation is valid for laminar flow
   b. At Reynolds numbers >2000, flow is likely to be turbulent
   c. Critical velocity is velocity above which flow of a fluid changes from turbulent to laminar
   d. In a narrow long tube, flow is likely to be laminar

385. Regarding the adjustable pressure limiting (APL) valve in the circle system on the modern anesthesia workstation, the *correct* statement is:
   a. The maximum pressure in the circle system allowed by the APL valve is 35 cm H_2O
   b. APL valve is best positioned between the patient and the inspiratory unidirectional valve
   c. It does not allow venting of fresh gases
   d. Heidbrink valve is an APL valve

386. Regarding humidification of inspired gas, the only *incorrect* statement is:
   a. At body temperature, fully heated and saturated inspired gas has an absolute humidity of 44 g m^{-3}
   b. Deposition of water droplets in the proximal airways is a common problem with ultrasonic nebulizers
   c. Heat moisture exchangers function poorly at high minute volumes (>10 litre/min) and at low patient temperatures
   d. Bubble humidifiers can achieve an absolute humidity of around 10–20 mg/L

387. Regarding nebulization and the likely behavior of water droplets of various sizes, the *incorrect* statement is:
   a. Droplets of 2–5 µm will be deposited within the bronchial tree
   b. Droplets of 0.5–1 µm will be deposited within the alveoli
   c. Droplets of >5 µm will be deposited within the main airways
   d. Droplets of <0.5 µm vaporize and do not reach the airways

388. Which of the following is not a electrical technique of measuring temperature?
   a. Compliance thermometer
   b. Thermocouple
   c. Resistance thermometer
   d. Thermistor

389. With reference to solubility coefficients in oil of inhaled anesthetics, the *correct* order is:
   a. Nitrous oxide > desflurane > Sevoflurane > Isoflurane
   b. Isoflurane > sevoflurane > desflurane > nitrous oxide
   c. Sevoflurane > isoflurane > desflurane > nitrous oxide
   d. Desflurane > nitrous oxide > sevoflurane > isoflurane

390. Laws or principles of physics have been paired with their examples or applications. Choose the *incorrect* pair:
   a. Daltons law of partial pressures : Fink effect
   b. Charles law : Calculating oxygen content of a pressurized oxygen cylinder
   c. Venturi effect : Jet nebulizer
   d. Avogadro's hypothesis : Calculating amount of gas in a nitrous oxide cylinder

391. What is *incorrect* about the ABO blood groups:
   a. Person of group O is a universal recipient
   b. A person of group A always has anti-B agglutinins in his plasma
   c. Donor cells are lysed by recipient antibodies in an incompatible blood transfusion reaction
   d. Disseminated intravascular coagulation may be a clue to mismatched transfusion

392. Compared with intracellular fluid, extracellular fluid has:
   a. Higher osmolarity
   b. Lower hydrogen ion concentration
   c. Lower chloride ion concentration
   d. Higher protein concentration

393. What is *incorrect* regarding pH and ionic dissociation?
   a. A weak acid will be 1000 times more ionized at a pH of 7 than at a pH of 4
   b. A strong alkali will have a high pH
   c. The pH is inversely proportional to the hydrogen ion concentration
   d. A pH of 7.7 corresponds to a hydrogen ion concentration of 20 nmol/L

394. What is *incorrect* concerning acid-base balance?
   a. Metabolic acidosis is seen with prolonged use of loop diuretics
   b. Standard bicarbonate is low in metabolic acidosis
   c. About 70% of carbon dioxide is transported in plasma as bicarbonate
   d. The ratio of HCO_3/CO_2 may be normal in a stable COPD patient

395. What is *incorrect* about adenyl cyclase?
   a. It catalyzes the conversion of ATP to cyclic AMP
   b. It is linked to stimulatory and inhibitory G proteins
   c. It is decreased by aminophylline
   d. It is an integral part of beta-adrenergic receptors

396. What is *correct* concerning bilirubin?
   a. A conjugated bilirubin of 20 mmol/L in a neonate will cause brain damage

b. The serum-conjugated bilirubin is increased in hemolysis
c. Barbiturates may be used to treat hyperbilirubinemia
d. Urinary urobilinogen excretion is decreased in obstructive jaundice

397. **Starvation initially causes:**
    a. Increase in serum glucose
    b. Increase in urinary nitrogen excretion
    c. Increase in glucose utilization by the brain
    d. Metabolic alkalosis

398. **Blood urea nitrogen is not increased in:**
    a. Gastrointestinal hemorrhage
    b. Excessive protein intake
    c. Dehydration
    d. End-stage liver disease

399. **Which of the following is a 39-residue hormone of the anterior pituitary gland?**
    a. Glucagon   b. Bradykinin
    c. Corticotropin   d. Insulin

400. **Which of the following enzyme is used in PCR?**
    a. EcoRII
    b. EcoRI
    c. Taq DNA polymerase
    d. HRP

401. **The number of milligrams of KOH required to neutralize the free and combined fatty acid in one gram of a given fat is called:**
    a. Polenske number
    b. Acid number
    c. Saponification number
    d. Iodine number

402. **Which of the following enzyme's activity is increased whenever the cell's ATP supply is depleted?**
    a. Pyruvate kinase
    b. Phosphofructokinase-1
    c. Hexokinase
    d. Glucokinase

403. **Which is the major factor determining whether glucose is oxidized by aerobic or anaerobic glycolysis?**
    a. Presence of high AMP
    b. NADH and the ATP/ADP ratio
    c. Ca^{+2}
    d. $FADH_2$

404. **Which of the following is the first amino group entering into urea cycle?**
    a. Arginine   b. Citrulline
    c. Carbamoyl phosphate   d. Ornithine

405. **Oxidation of which substance in the body yields the most calories?**
    a. Glucose   b. Glycogen
    c. Protein   d. Lipids

406. **The exchange of material across cell membrane takes place:**
    a. Only by diffusion
    b. Only by active transport
    c. Only by pinocytosis
    d. All of these

407. **The pH of blood is 7.4 when the ratio between H_2CO_3 and $NaHCO_3$ is:**
    a. 1:10   b. 1:20
    c. 1:25   d. 1:30

408. **Compounds having the same structural formula but differing in spatial configuration are known as:**
    a. Stereoisomers
    b. Anomers
    c. Optical isomers
    d. Epimers

409. **Which of the following does not give a positive Benedict's test?**
    a. Sucrose   b. Lactose
    c. Maltose   d. Glucose

410. **Starch is a:**
    a. Polysaccharide
    b. Monosaccharide
    c. Disaccharide
    d. None of these

411. **A carbohydrate, commonly known as dextrose is:**
    a. Dextrin
    b. D-Fructose
    c. D-Sucrose
    d. Glycogen

412. **In which of the following conditions, the specific gravity of urine increases?**
    a. Diabetes mellitus
    b. Chronic glomerulonephritis
    c. Compulsive polydypsia
    d. Hypercalcemia

413. **Lactate formed in muscles can be utilized through which cycle?**
    a. Rapoport-Luebeling cycle
    b. Glucose-alanine cycle
    c. Cori's cycle
    d. Citric acid cycle

414. **In which group of the following organs, Glucose-6-phosphatase is not present?**
    a. Liver and kidneys

b. Kidneys and muscles
c. Kidneys and adipose tissue
d. Muscles and adipose tissue

415. Gluconeogenesis is decreased by:
    a. Glucagon
    b. Epinephrine
    c. Glucocorticoids
    d. Insulin

416. What is the function of Cori's cycle? It transfers:
    a. Glucose from muscles to liver
    b. Lactate from muscles to liver
    c. Lactate from liver to muscles
    d. Pyruvate from liver to muscles

417. During starvation, ketone bodies are used as a fuel by:
    a. Erythrocytes
    b. Brain
    c. Liver
    d. All of these

418. In the diet of a diabetic patient, the recommended carbohydrate intake should preferably be in the form of:
    a. Monosaccharides
    b. Disaccharides
    c. Polysaccharides
    d. All of these

419. The conversion of alanine to glucose is known as:
    a. Glycolysis
    b. Oxidative decarboxylation
    c. Specific dynamic action
    d. Gluconeogenesis

420. How many moles of ATPs are generated from one mole of glucose by glycolysis under anaerobic conditions?
    a. One
    b. Two
    c. Eight
    d. Thirty

421. Which of the following enzymes is required for glycolysis?
    a. Pyruvate kinase
    b. Pyruvate carboxylase
    c. Glucose-6-phosphatase
    d. Glycerokinase

422. Which of the following molecule does not give positive Rothera's test result?
    a. β-hydroxy butyrate
    b. Acetone
    c. Acetoacetic acid
    d. b + c

423. Statins act on which step of cholesterol biosynthesis?
    a. Selective competitive inhibitor of HMG-CoA reductase
    b. Selective competitive inhibitor of HMG-CoA synthase
    c. Selective non-competitive inhibitor of HMG-CoA reductase
    d. Selective non-competitive inhibitor of HMG-CoA synthase

424. Which of the following conditions result in increased gluconeogenesis?
    a. Diabetes mellitus and atherosclerosis
    b. Fed condition and thyrotoxicosis
    c. Diabetes mellitus and starvation
    d. Alcohol intake and cigarette smoking

425. Which of the following statements regarding the glucose absorption in the digestive tract is most appropriate?
    a. It occurs in the small intestine
    b. It is stimulated by the hormone glucagon
    c. It occurs more rapidly than the absorption of any other sugar
    d. It is impaired in cases of diabetes mellitus

426. Most of the metabolic pathways are either anabolic or catabolic. Which of the following pathways is considered as "amphibolic" in nature?
    a. Glycogenesis
    b. Glycolytic pathway
    c. Lipolysis
    d. Kreb's cycle

427. During the normal resting state of humans, most of the blood glucose burnt as "fuel" is consumed by:
    a. Liver
    b. Brain
    c. Kidneys
    d. Adipose tissue

428. Major histocompatibility (MHC) proteins are unique to:
    a. Each cell
    b. Each organ
    c. Each individual
    d. Each species

429. Which of the following reserve nutrient gets depleted the first during starvation?
    a. Glycogen
    b. Proteins
    c. Triglycerides
    d. Cholesterol

430. In hypoparathyroidism:
    a. Plasma calcium and inorganic phosphorous are low
    b. Plasma calcium and inorganic phosphorous are high
    c. Plasma calcium is low and inorganic phosphorous high
    d. Plasma calcium is high and inorganic phosphorous low

431. Which of the following is the most sensitive indicator of glomerular function?
    a. Serum urea
    b. Serum creatinine
    c. Urea clearance
    d. Creatinine clearance

432. Which one of the following is a test of tubular function?
    a. Creatinine clearance
    b. Inulin clearance
    c. Para-aminohippurate (PAH) clearance
    d. Urine osmolality

433. What is GABA (gama amino butyric acid)?
    a. Post-synaptic excitatory transmitter
    b. Post-synaptic inhibitor transmitter
    c. Activator of glia-cell function
    d. Inhibitor of glia-cell function

434. Which is the major end waste product of protein nitrogen metabolism in human?
    a. Glycine
    b. Uric acid
    c. Urea
    d. Ammonia

435. How is ammonia is efficiently cleared from brain?
    a. Creatinine formation
    b. Urea production
    c. Uric acid formation
    d. Glutamine formation

436. Which one of the following is an essential amino acid?
    a. Arginine
    b. Tyrosine
    c. Phenylalanine
    d. Proline

437. Which one of the following condition can be a cause of hemolytic jaundice?
    a. G-6 phosphatase deficiency
    b. Increased conjugated bilirubin
    c. Glucokinase deficiency
    d. Phosphoglucomutase deficiency

438. In which of the condition, increase in fecal urobilinogen is observed?
    a. Hemolytic jaundice
    b. Obstruction of biliary duct
    c. Extrahepatic gallstones
    d. Enlarged lymph nodes

439. Hepatocellular jaundice as compared to pure obstructive type of jaundice is characterized by:
    a. Increased serum alkaline phosphate, LDH and ALT
    b. Decreased serum alkaline phosphatase, LDH and ALT
    c. Increased serum alkaline phosphatase and decreased levels of LDH and ALT
    d. Decreased serum alkaline phosphatase and increased serum LDH and ALT

440. Daily protein requirement of an adult woman is:
    a. 0.5 gm/kg of body weight
    b. 0.8 gm/kg of body weight
    c. 1.0 gm/kg of body weight
    d. 1.5 gm/kg of body weight

441. In which of the following conditions, bile pigments are absent and urobilinogen increased in urine?
    a. Hemolytic jaundice
    b. Hepatocellular jaundice
    c. Obstructive jaundice
    d. Rotor's syndrome

442. Prothrombin is synthesized in:
    a. Erythrocytes
    b. Reticulo-endothelial cells
    c. Liver
    d. Kidneys

443. In which of the following conditions, prothrombin time will remain prolonged even after parenteral administration of vitamin K?
    a. Hemolytic jaundice
    b. Ischemic hepatitis
    c. Biliary obstruction
    d. Steatorrhea

444. Prostaglandins are synthesized in the body from:
    a. Linolenic acid
    b. Arachidonic acid
    c. Stearic acid
    d. Linoleic acid

445. Which one of the following is *correct* statement regarding the process of non-shivering thermogenesis?
    a. Glucose is oxidized to lactate
    b. Fatty acids uncouple oxidative phosphorylation
    c. Ethanol is formed
    d. ATP is burned for heat production

446. Which enzyme rises the earliest following myocardial infarction?
    a. Creatine kinase
    b. GOT
    c. GPT
    d. LDH

447. Carbonic anhydrase is competitively inhibited by:
    a. Allopurinol
    b. Acetazolamide
    c. Aminopterin
    d. Neostigmine

448. Glucose is the only source of energy for:
    a. Myocardium
    b. Kidneys
    c. Erythrocytes
    d. Thrombocytes

449. Which one of the following facts is most appropriate regarding a coenzyme?
    a. It is often a vitamin
    b. Is is always an inorganic compound
    c. It is always a protein
    d. It is often a metal compound

450. According to recommendations for PONV management in adults, how many drugs should be given for PONV prophylaxis if patient has 1–2 risk factors?
    a. 4
    b. 3
    c. 2
    d. 1

451. As per Indian guidelines on nutrition in critically ill patient, which statement does not indicate gut dysfunction?
    a. Regurgitation/Vomiting
    b. Aspiration (feeding formula in tracheal aspirate)
    c. Gastric residual volume > 300 mL (monitoring 4–8 hrs)
    d. 1–2 loose stools/day

452. According to the ISCCM guidelines for antibiotics therapy in immunocompromised patients, which statement is not *true* for vancomycin?
    a. It is effective against MRSA
    b. It is effective for blood infection showing gram negative bacilli
    c. It is used in soft tissue infection
    d. It can be considered in severe mucositis

453. According to the ISCCM guidelines for antibiotics therapy in immunocompromised patients which statement is *correct*?
    a. One blood culture is enough to establish diagnosis
    b. At least 5 mL of blood is required for culture
    c. Central venous line culture is not necessary
    d. In case of multi-lumen catheter, one set per lumen should be collected

454. According to ASRA guidelines for treatment of local anesthesia toxicity (LAST) what is the maximum dose of Intra-lipid which can be used?
    a. 10 mL/kg
    b. 12 mL/kg
    c. 15 mL/kg
    d. 1.5 mL/kg

455. Which of the following drugs does not increase hypoxic pulmonary vascular resistance?
    a. Beta adrenergic receptor blockers
    b. Alpha adrenergic receptor agonists
    c. Cyclooxygenase inhibitors
    d. ACE inhibitors

456. Which factor causes the oxygen dissociation curve to shift to the right?
    a. Decreased temperature
    b. Decreased 2,3 DPG
    c. Increased hydrogen ions
    d. Decreased $PaCO_2$

457. At what partial pressure of oxygen (PaO_2), do chemoreceptors stimulate breathing?
    a. 80 mm Hg
    b. 70 mm Hg
    c. 60 mm Hg
    d. None of the above

458. QT interval includes:
    a. Ventricular depolarization
    b. Ventricular repolarization
    c. Both depolarization and repolarization
    d. Atrial depolarization and repolarization

459. What is the basal rate of insulin secretion in portal venous system?
    a. 2 IU/hr
    b. 3 IU/hr
    c. 1 IU/hr
    d. 0.5 IU/hr

460. Which of the following is the side effect of cisplatin chemotherapy?
    a. Ototoxicity
    b. Renal toxicity
    c. Neuropathy
    d. All of the above

461. Muscle relaxants metabolized by butyryl cholinesterase?
    a. Vecuronium
    b. Cistaracurium
    c. Atracurium
    d. Mivacurium

462. What are the sizes of three lumens of the central line of size 7 Fr?
    a. 16,18,18 G
    b. 14,16,18 G
    c. 14,18,18 G
    d. 14, 16,16 G

463. Which statement is *true* regarding vascular catheters?
    a. Flow is inversely proportional to the radius of the catheter
    b. Flow is inversely proportional to the length of the catheter

c. Flow is directly proportional to the radius and the length of the catheter
d. Flow is inversely proportional to the radius and the length of the catheter

464. **ARISCAT scoring is used for:**
    a. Predict postoperative pulmonary complications
    b. Prediction of surgical complications
    c. Used for deep vein thrombosis
    d. Score for predicting postoperative hepatic failure

465. **Nine panel plot is used for interpretation of:**
    a. Cardiopulmonary exercise test
    b. Arterial blood gas analysis
    c. Spirometry
    d. Comparison of several clinical or scientific studies studying the same thing

466. **Inferior mediastinum is subdivided into:**
    a. Anterior and posterior
    b. Anterior, middle and posterior
    c. Anterior and middle
    d. Middle and posterior mediastinum

467. **Which are the constituents of EMLA cream?**
    a. 2.5% Lignocaine + 2.5% Prilocaine
    b. 4% Lignocaine + 1% Prilocaine
    c. 3% Lignocaine + 2% Prilocaine
    d. 2% Lignocaine + 2% Prilocaine

468. **Which size is not available in double lumen tube (DLT)?**
    a. 26 Fr
    b. 28 Fr
    c. 30 Fr
    d. 32 Fr

469. **Which of the following hemodynamic change is not associated with Pringle's maneuver during hepatic resection?**
    a. An increase in systemic vascular resistance
    b. Increase in blood pressure
    c. Decreased cardiac output
    d. Decrease in blood pressure

470. **Which are the Vitamin K dependent factors?**
    a. II, III, VIII, IX
    b. II, VII, IX, X
    c. III, VII, VIII, X
    d. II, IX, X, XI

471. **Which is the most common neuropathy in lithotomy position?**
    a. Common peroneal nerve
    b. Femoral nerve
    c. Popliteal nerve
    d. Sciatic nerve

472. **Which of the following statement regarding coagulation is *incorrect*?**
    a. Prothrombin time (PT) represents integrity of intrinsic and common pathways
    b. aPTT represents integrity of intrinsic and common pathways
    c. Antiphospholipid antibodies can prolong PT
    d. Polycythemia with hematocrit >55 can lead to false high PT

473. **Total score in modified Aldrete criteria is:**
    a. 8   b. 6
    c. 10   d. 12

474. **What does 'a" wave in CVP represent?**
    a. Atrial contraction
    b. Atrial relaxation
    c. Ventricular contraction
    d. Ventricular relaxation

475. **Tuffier's line is at the following level till infancy?**
    a. L3–L4
    b. L4–L5
    c. L5–S1
    d. L2–L3

476. **Sacral hiatus is formed due to lack of fusion of which vertebrae?**
    a. Fifth and fourth sacral vertebrae
    b. Fifth and sixth sacral vertebrae
    c. Third and fourth sacral vertebrae
    d. Second and third sacral vertebrae

477. **Regarding emergence delirium in children, which of the following statement is not *correct*?**
    a. Sevoflurane causes more emergence delirium than halothane
    b. PAED score >10 is considered as emergence delirium
    c. Incidence is higher in patients between the ages of 2 and 6
    d. Watcha scale is a better predictor than PAED scale

478. **Which of the following glomerular disease is known to have a 100% recurrence rate after kidney transplant?**
    a. Dense deposit disease (DDD)
    b. Focal segmental glomerulosclerosis
    c. Membranous glomerulonephritis
    d. Membrano proliferative glomerulonephritis

479. **Which of the following analgesic is to be avoided after renal transplantation?**
    a. Fentanyl
    b. Paracetamol
    c. Hydrocodone
    d. Meperidine

480. Which of the following is not *true* regarding brain-stem death?
    a. Absence of spontaneous respiration
    b. Presence of doll's eye movement
    c. Absence of gag reflex
    d. Absence of eye movements on caloric testing

481. Which of the following is *true* regarding anesthesia management for beating brain dead organ donation?
    a. High tidal volume ventilation to target $PO_2 > 300$
    b. Maintenance of hypothermia
    c. Syndrome of inappropriate antidiuretic hormone secretion (SIADH) requiring vasopressin infusion
    d. Hormone cocktail containing thyroxine, insulin, steroids and vasopressin may be required in some cases

482. The Milan criteria is used for selecting:
    a. Patients with end stage renal disease for kidney transplant
    b. Patients with heart failure for cardiac transplant
    c. Patients with primary liver tumors for liver transplant
    d. Patients with interstitial lung disease for lung transplant

483. Fluid responsiveness is defined by:
    a. Increase in blood pressure
    b. Decrease in heart rate
    c. Increase in central venous pressure
    d. Increase in stroke volume

484. Which of the following is not an intervention for inadequate cerebral perfusion pressure:
    a. Reduce brain edema
    b. Remove cerebrospinal fluid
    c. Increase cerebral metabolic rate ($CMRO_2$)
    d. Increase mean arterial pressure

485. Which of the following is not feature of cirrhotic cardiomyopathy?
    a. Systolic and diastolic dysfunction
    b. Reduced contractile reserve
    c. Shortened QT interval
    d. Reduced exercise tolerance

486. Which of the following agent should be avoided in neurosurgeries:
    a. Dexamethasone
    b. Dexmedetomidine
    c. Remifentanil
    d. Nitrous oxide

487. Which type of dyspnea is unique in patients with hepatopulmonary (HPS) syndrome?
    a. Dyspnea
    b. Trepopnea
    c. Orthopnea
    d. Platypnea

488. Which of the following is not *true* regarding lung transplant:
    a. Single lung transplant is technically simpler
    b. Patients with interstitial lung disease can benefit with single lung transplant
    c. Patients with pulmonary artery hypertension benefit with single lung transplant
    d. Bilateral lung transplant accounts for 80% of all the lung transplant

489. Post-reperfusion syndrome (PRS) is a significant event and can lead to arrhythmias and even cardiac arrest, in which phase of liver transplant?
    a. Anhepatic phase
    b. Neohepatic phase
    c. Pre-anhepatic phase
    d. Can occur in any of the above phases

490. Which of the following statement is *false* regarding cerebral blood flow?
    a. Blood flow to the brain is through internal carotid and vertebral arteries
    b. The anterior and posterior circulations anastomose at the base of the brain to form Circle of Willis
    c. The Circle of Willis may be incomplete in 50% of individuals
    d. About 50% of the cerebral flow is by the internal carotid artery

491. Which of the following is not an effect of Phenylephrine?
    a. Alpha 1 agonist
    b. Pulmonary vasoconstriction
    c. Reflex tachycardia
    d. Increase in systemic blood pressure

492. Which is the functional unit of the liver?
    a. Lobule   b. Porta hepatis
    c. Acinus   d. Portal triad

493. Which of the following is not used to differentiate between standard and extended criteria donors?
    a. Age   b. Diabetes mellitus
    c. Hypertension   d. Serum creatinine

494. Which of the following statement is *correct*?
    a. Fospropofol has immediate onset of action
    b. Dexmedetomidine can cause significant respiratory depression
    c. Remimazolam has organ independent elimination
    d. Methoxycarbonyletomidate (MOC-etomidate) has a longer half-life than etomidate

495. Which of the following immunosuppresant is an *incorrect* match?
    a. Sirolimus—Calcineurin inhibitor
    b. Cyclophosphamide—Antimetabolite

c. Basiliximab—Monoclonal antibody
d. Mycophenolate mofetil—Antimetabolite

496. **Which of the following is primarily responsible for thermoregulation?**
    a. Thalamus
    b. Spinothalamic tract
    c. Hypothalamus
    d. Pons

497. **Which of the following is *false* regarding temperature management during anesthesia?**
    a. General anesthesia increases the shivering threshold
    b. Radiation is the major method of heat loss under Anesthesia
    c. Meperidine and dexmedetomidine can be used to treat shivering
    d. Hypothermia can cause coagulation defects

498. **Pertaining to ABO blood groups, which is the best *correct* statement?**
    a. The most common blood group is B
    b. Type B blood has Anti-A antibodies in the plasma
    c. Type O can be safely transfused to anyone without risk of transfusion reactions
    d. Crossmatch involves mixing the donor plasma with recipient's red blood cells and checking for agglutination

499. **Which statement is *correct* about morphine?**
    a. High lipid solubility
    b. 80% bound to plasma proteins
    c. Metabolized by conjugation in the liver
    d. Metabolite morphine-3-glucuronide is more potent μ-receptor agonist and contributes to morphine's analgesic effects

500. **Which condition shifts the Oxyhemoglobin dissociation curve to the left?**
    a. Acidosis
    b. Pregnancy
    c. Carbon monoxide poisoning
    d. Acclimatization at high altitudes

501. **In geriatric patients:**
    a. Body water is increased
    b. Closing capacity is increased
    c. Functional residual capacity (FRC) is decreased
    d. Creatinine clearance remains normal

502. **Stress response results in the following endocrine changes:**
    a. Decreased glucagon secretion
    b. ACTH secretion is decreased
    c. ADH secretion is increased
    d. Growth hormone secretion is decreased

503. **Which of the following is a paramagnetic gas?**
    a. Nitrous oxide
    b. Carbon dioxide
    c. Oxygen
    d. Sevoflurane

504. **Which of the following statements is *true* regarding a T-piece?**
    a. Can be used only in pediatric patients
    b. Is a Mapleson E with an open ended reservoir bag
    c. Is an efficient system
    d. With a constant fresh gas flow, a small reservoir has no effect on the performance of the system

505. **The emergency O_2 flush on an anesthesia machine:**
    a. Delivers O_2 at 20 litres/min
    b. Is safe to use during anesthesia
    c. Can be safely used with a minute volume divider ventilator
    d. Increases the risk of awareness during anesthesia

506. **Which statement is *true* regarding the desflurane Tec 6 vaporizer?**
    a. Desflurane is heated to a temperature of 30°C
    b. The vaporization chamber is pressurized to 1550 mmHg (approx 2 bar)
    c. The percentage control dial calibration is from 0–8%
    d. Requires a special adaptor to allow mounting on the Selectatec system

507. **A high pulmonary capillary wedge pressure (PCWP) is seen in:**
    a. Pulmonary hypertension
    b. Pulmonary embolism
    c. Left ventricular failure
    d. Tricuspid regurgitation

508. **Choose *correct* option:**
    In neuromuscular monitoring:
    a. The nerve stimulator should be able to produce a constant voltage for a variety of currents and impedance
    b. A double burst stimulation lasts less than 0.1 ms
    c. A double burst stimulation is more accurate but more difficult to detect visually then TOF
    d. For accurate mechanomyography, a preload of 100–300 g must be applied

509. **Choose the best *correct* option**
    As per fasting guidelines,
    a. Clear fluids will empty from an adult stomach in 3 - 4 hours
    b. Solids will usually empty from the stomach in 8 hours
    c. Milk empties from the stomach at the same rate as other fluids
    d. Recommend a minimum fast of 4 hours for breast milk

510. **Choose the *correct* option Pertaining to breathing circuits,**
    a. Mapleson B is used as a co-axial circuit
    b. Mapleson D circuits are more efficient for spontaneous ventilation
    c. Flows with the Ayres T piece should be 1.5 times the patient's minute volume for spontaneous respiration
    d. The Lack circuit is more efficient for spontaneous ventilation than controlled ventilation

511. **Which statement is *true* regarding malignant hyperthermia during anesthesia?**
    a. Sevoflurane does not precipitate
    b. Inheritance is by an autosomal dominant mechanism
    c. Mannitol is added to vials of dantrolene for management of haemoglobinuria
    d. Profound muscle weakness can result from the effect of dantrolene on calcium transport

512. **Which statement is *true* regarding physiological changes in pregnancy?**
    a. An increase in cardiac output mainly due to an increase in heart rate
    b. Increase in minute ventilation is caused by increase in tidal volume
    c. Gastric acidity increases in the third trimester
    d. Gastric emptying is delayed in pregnancy

513. **What is *true* about the epidural catheters?**
    a. At least 10 cm of the catheter should be inserted into an adult epidural space
    b. The catheter should not be withdrawn through the Touhy needle once it has been threaded beyond the bevel
    c. Catheters with a single port at the distal tip reduce incidence of vascular or dural puncture
    d. The catheters are not radio-opaque

514. **Which is the *correct* property of Fentanyl?**
    a. Has a potency 10 times that of Morphine
    b. Is lipid soluble
    c. Does not accumulate despite repeated boluses
    d. Is metabolised to an active metabolite, norfentanyl

515. **Total cerebral blood flow in humans is:**
    a. Approximately 15% of the resting cardiac output
    b. Reduced significantly if the mean arterial pressure is reduced from 120 mm Hg to 80 mm Hg
    c. Regulated by sympathetic nerves from the cervical sympathetic chain
    d. Increased during intense mental activity

516. **Pertaining to Post dural puncture headache (PDPH):**
    a. Yale and Quincke needle designs have a lower incidence of PDPH
    b. PDPH is inversely proportional to the size of the needle used
    c. The incidence of PDPH is similar in young and elderly population
    d. It is proportional to the number of dural punctures

517. **Choose the best *correct* option**
    Cerebral blood flow is:
    a. Increased by an increase in carbon dioxide concentration in the arterial blood
    b. Reduced significantly if the mean systemic blood pressure is reduced from 120 mm Hg to 80 mm Hg
    c. Regulated by sympathetic nerves from the cervical sympathetic chain
    d. Increased during intense mental activity

518. **Laminar flow through a tube is:**
    a. Proportional to its density
    b. Proportional to the square of its radius
    c. Directly proportional to the length of the tube
    d. Inversely proportional to the viscosity

519. **Fetal hemoglobin (HbF):**
    a. Makes up 80% hemoglobin at birth
    b. Consists of two alpha and two delta chains
    c. Makes up 20% of hemoglobin at 6 months of age
    d. Has lower affinity for oxygen in comparison with adult hemoglobin (HbA)

520. **During an epidural catheter insertion, cerebrospinal fluid can be identified in a suspected dural puncture in the following way:**
    a. Forms a cloudy precipitate with levobupivacaine
    b. Turns litmus paper pink
    c. Is straw colored
    d. Forms a cloudy precipitate with thiopentone

521. **About the carotid body:**
    a. It consists of stretch receptors
    b. Receives blood supply, four times that of the brain
    c. Stimulated by decrease in pH
    d. Stimulated by carbon monoxide poisoning

522. **During a valsalva manoeuvre:**
    a. There is an initial fall in blood pressure at the start of straining
    b. Associated with bradycardia during the manoeuvre
    c. Stimulates baroreceptors
    d. There is an increase in intracranial pressure

523. **Which of the following is a parasympathetic ganglion?**
    a. The stellate ganglion
    b. The gasserian ganglion
    c. The celiac ganglion
    d. The ciliary ganglion

524. **Q-T interval on an ECG:**
    a. Represents the duration of the ventricular diastole
    b. Measured from end of the QRS complex to the end of the T wave
    c. Shortened in hypokalemia, hypothermia and hypocalcemia and digoxin therapy
    d. Prolonged QT is associated with recurrent syncope or sudden death due to ventricular arrhythmias including Torsade de pointes

525. **Regarding Allen's test:**
    a. Originally described for assessing arterial flow to the hand in thromboangiitis obliterans
    b. Used for assessing radial artery flow prior to radial arterial cannulation
    c. Return of the color of the hand in less than 10-20 seconds, is considered normal
    d. Though widely performed, may be inaccurate in predicting risk from ischemic damage

526. **What is *true* about oxygen concentrators:**
    a. They concentrate oxygen that has been delivered from an oxygen cylinder manifold
    b. Argon can accumulate when oxygen concentrators are used with a circle system
    c. They can achieve oxygen concentrations of up to 100%
    d. Can be used only in home oxygen therapy

527. **The brachial plexus is formed due to fusion of:**
    a. The ventral primary rami of cervical nerves 5 to 8 and first thoracic nerve (C5-T1), including a greater part of the second thoracic nerve (T2)
    b. The ventral primary rami of cervical nerves 5 to 8 (C5-C8), including a greater part of the first thoracic nerve (T1)
    c. The dorsal primary rami of cervical nerves 5 to 8 and first thoracic nerve (C5-T1), including a greater part of the second thoracic nerve (T2)
    d. The dorsal primary rami of cervical nerves 5 to 8 (C5-C8), including a greater part of the first thoracic nerve (T1). 59

528. **What constitutes the medial cord of brachial plexus?**
    a. The anterior division of the middle and inferior trunk
    b. The anterior division of the inferior trunk
    c. The anterior division of the superior and middle trunk
    d. The anterior division of the middle trunk

529. **With respect to the brachial plexus, the trunks divide into divisions (anterior and posterior)**
    a. At the inter scalene grove, between the anterior and middle scalene muscles
    b. At the exit of the axilla
    c. At the lateral border of the first rib, behind the clavicle
    d. In the axilla with reference to the second part of the axillary artery

530. **With respect to principles of brachial plexus block, which of the following statements is *true*?**
    a. In the supraclavicular approach, the trunks and divisions of the plexus is blocked providing the most widespread surgical anesthesia for the whole arm
    b. In the supraclavicular approach, the trunks and divisions of the plexus is blocked providing anesthesia for elbow, forearm and hand
    c. In the supraclavicular approach, the cords of the plexus is blocked providing the most widespread surgical anesthesia for the whole arm
    d. In the supraclavicular approach, the cords of the plexus is blocked providing the most widespread surgical anesthesia for elbow, forearm and hand

531. **The nerve that arises from the trunk of brachial plexus is:**
    a. Long thoracic nerve
    b. Dorsal scapular nerve
    c. Lateral pectoral nerve
    d. Suprascapular nerve

532. **Which of the following is not associated with increased risk of ocular penetration and perforation during ophthalmic blocks?**
    a. Myopia with staphyloma
    b. Patients with prior scleral buckle procedure
    c. Enophthalmos
    d. Elderly

533. **Which of the following statement is *true* with respect to retro bulbar blocks?**
    a. The LA is injected behind the eye and outside the muscle cone
    b. Larger volume of LA is needed for quick onset of the block
    c. Conjunctival chemosis is less than peribulbar block
    d. The incidence of serious complication like hematoma, scleral perforation, oculocardaiac reflex is less compared to subtenons block

534. **Which of the following statement is *true* with respect to sub- Tenon's blocks?**
    a. This is also known as subscleral block
    b. This block is not preferred in the western world
    c. It is associated with inherent risks of needle-based blocks like perforation of eyeball and optic nerve damage
    d. It is also effective in strabismus surgeries

535. With respect to ultrasound blocks for the eye—which of the following statement is *true*?
    a. Ultrasound guided ophthalmic blocks is technically challenging as the orbit is not well suited for ultrasound examination
    b. Excessive sound energy can cause mechanical and thermal damage to the eye
    c. Linear transducers used for peripheral blocks are most suitable for eye blocks
    d. The spread of the local anesthetic to produce an optic perineural 'V' sign has significant correlation with block success

536. In the original technique for Biers block the local anesthetic used was:
    a. Lidocaine
    b. Procaine
    c. Cocaine
    d. Prilocaine

537. Which of the following is not a contraindication for Biers block?
    a. Lymphoedema
    b. Procedure needed in both arms
    c. Uncooperative or confused patients
    d. Anemia

538. Pk_a value of lidocaine in aqueous solution is:
    a. 7.7
    b. 7.8
    c. 8.1
    d. 8.0

539. With respect to conduction blocking potency of local anesthetics, which of the following local anesthetic belongs to high potency?
    a. Lidocaine
    b. Chlorprocaine
    c. Bupivacaine
    d. Mepivacaine

540. Following which of the blocks, the longest duration of local anesthetic effect of a single bolus dose is seen?
    a. Lumbar plexus block
    b. Transversus abdominis block
    c. Brachial plexus block
    d. Intrathecal block

541. During Tumescent anesthesia, the total dose of lidocaine used to produce safe plasma concentration is:
    a. 5–7 mg/kg of lidocaine with adrenaline
    b. 5–7 mg/kg of lidocaine without adrenaline
    c. 15–25 mg/kg of lidocaine with adrenaline
    d. 35 to 55 mg/kg of lidocaine with adrenaline

542. With respect to the various routes of administration of local anesthetic, systemic absorption is the highest after
    a. Intercostal nerve blockade
    b. Caudal epidural space
    c. Lumbar epidural space
    d. Subcutaneous tissue

543. With respect to toxicity and allergies associated with local anesthetics, which of the following statement is *true*?
    a. Development of methemoglobinemia is a unique side effect associated with administration of large dose of procaine
    b. The potential for toxicity with lidocaine infusions is increased in neonates due to accumulation of its principal metabolite glycylxylidide (GX), which can cause seizures
    c. It is not recommended that bupivacaine induced ventricular arrhythmia be treated with lidocaine or amiodarone
    d. Aminoamide local anesthetic are associated more commonly with allergic type of reactions

544. Though the pathophysiology of post-dural puncture headache (PDPH) is not completely established, which of the following is not a likely to contribute to PDPH?
    a. The CSF volume loss causes a downward pull of pain sensitive structures leading to PDPH
    b. Concentration of substance P and regulation of neurokinin 1 receptor is responsible for PDPH
    c. The dural puncture allows CSF to leak leading to decreased CSF volume and pressure which contributes to PDPH
    d. Loss of CSF flow leads to compensatory venous vasoconstriction which adds to symptoms of PDPH

545. Which of the following needle is not an 'atraumatic' spinal needle?
    a. Whitacre
    b. Quincke
    c. Sprotte
    d. Atraucan

546. Which the following statements is *true* with respect to post-dural puncture headache (PDPH)?
    a. The incidence of PDPH after unintentional dural puncture during labor analgesia is 20–30%
    b. Blood patch is an effective prophylactic measure to reduce PDPH
    c. In 90% of the cases the headache starts within 72 hours of the dural puncture
    d. The epidural blood patch is the gold standard of treatment with complete relief of symptoms in 73% of patients

547. With respect to the spinal column and spinal nerves which of the following statement is *true*:
    a. Spinal nerve that exit the cord are numbered as thoracic, lumbar, sacral based on the vertebra above
    b. The spinal cord in adults ends at upper end of L1 vertebra
    c. The dural sac ends at upper border of S2
    d. 1–7 cervical nerves are numbered according to the vertebra above

548. Which nerves are blocked by complete scalp block?.
    a. Supraorbital, supratrochlear, zygomaticofacial, greater and lesser occipital nerves
    b. Supraorbital, supratrochlear, auriculotemporal, zygomaticotemporal, greater and lesser occipital nerves
    c. Supraorbital, supratrochlear, auriculotemporal, greater auricular, greater and lesser occipital nerves
    d. Supraorbital, supratrochlear, zygomaticofacial, greater auricular and lesser occipital nerves

549. Which of the following is not a branch form the superficial cervical plexus?
    a. Lesser occipital
    b. Greater occipital
    c. Transverse cervical
    d. Supraclavicular nerves

550. "Meralgia paresthetica" is a condition in which there exist sensory disturbance along the:
    a. Femoral nerve
    b. Obturator nerve
    c. Genitofemoral nerve
    d. Lateral femoral cutaneous nerve

551. Which of the following nerve arises form the sacral plexus?
    a. Genitofemoral nerve
    b. Saphenous nerve
    c. Pudendal nerve
    d. Ilioinguinal nerve

552. The trident sign during ultrasound of spine is related to:
    a. Acoustic shadows of the ribs
    b. Interlaminar spaces and adjoining laminae
    c. Acoustic shadows of the transverse process
    d. Superior articular processes and its acoustic shadow

553. Which of the following statements is *true* with respect to the femoral nerve block?
    a. The femoral nerve appears as a triangular hypoechoic area lateral to the artery using a high frequency linear probe
    b. The nerve is blocked best using an line plane technique and probe held in longitudinal axis over the inguinal crease
    c. The femoral sheath lies between the fascia lata and fascia iliaca, on the anterior aspect of the iliopsoas muscle
    d. During femoral block, depositing the local anesthetic only anteriorly to the nerve results in fewer needle redirection and greater satisfaction then depositing the drug circumferentially of the nerve

554. In patients admitted with fracture neck of femur, which block is recommended by Scottish Intercollegiate Guidelines Network?
    a. Femoral nerve block
    b. Fascia iliaca compartment block
    c. Lateral cutaneous nerve of the thigh
    d. Lumbar plexus nerve block

555. A strategy shown to reduce the incidence of severe phantom limb pain is the use of:
    a. Continuous regional analgesia using nerve sheath catheters
    b. Patient controlled analgesia with opioids post-operatively
    c. Preventive epidural analgesia using ketamine and local anaesthetic
    d. Perioperative gabapentinoids

556. Regarding epidural abcess, which statement is not *true*?
    a. Diagnosis is dependent on triad of back pain, fever, and paralysis
    b. Occurs at a rate of 1:1000–3000 (OR 1:2000 1:5000)
    c. Worse outcomes in advanced age
    d. Usually caused by gram positive cocci

557. Celiac plexus block is not effective in reducing pain originating from:
    a. Pancreas
    b. Transverse portion of the large colon
    c. Gallbladder
    d. Descending portion of the pelvic colon

558. Which rami form the brachial plexus?
    a. C5-T1 anterior primary
    b. C3-T2 anterior primary
    c. C5-T1 anterior and posterior
    d. C3-T2 anterior and posterior

559. A 60-year-old diabetic has had a above knee amputation for lower extremity sarcoma. He has neuropathic pain being managed with morphine 40 mg bd and paracetamol 1 gm qid. He is also on omeprazole 20 mg daily for reflux. You decide to commence gabapentin. Before deciding on a dosage regimen and commencing therapy it is most important that you:
    a. Cease his omeprazole

b. Check his hepatic transaminase level
c. Check his renal function
d. Check his QT interval on a resting EGG

560. Regarding complex regional pain syndrome, which statement is *true*?
a. Characterized by disabling pain, swelling, vasomotor instability, sudomotor abnormality, and impairment of motor function
b. Type II CRPS was formally known as reflex sympathetic dystrophy
c. To be managed with sympathetic blocks only
d. Physiotherapy has no role

561. Sympathetic block is not used in the following condition:
a. Reynaud's syndrome
b. Herpes zoster
c. Migraine
d. Bony metastasis

562. Which of the following is not a clinical feature of fibromyalgia?
a. Joint stiffness
b. Mood disorder
c. Sleep disturbance
d. Constipation

563. Which statement is *true* regarding management of fibromyalgia?
a. Educating the patient regarding the condition plays an important role
b. Tri-cyclic agents are not beneficial in treating pain
c. There is evidence that strong opioids are beneficial
d. There is evidence that steroids are beneficial

564. Most commonly missed nerve with interscalene approach to brachial plexus is:
a. Ulnar
b. Median
c. Musculocutaneous
d. Radial

565. Artery of Adamkiewicz arises at following spinal level:
a. T1–T6
b. T5–T8
c. T9–L2
d. T11–L3

566. Approaches to celiac plexus are all, *except*:
a. Anterocrural
b. Lateral
c. Transcrural
d. Retrocrural

567. Complete the statement with most appropriate answer:
McGill Pain Questionnaire:
a. Consists of three major measures to be assessed
b. Was developed by McGill
c. Is not widely used
d. Is a single-dimensional pain scale

568. "Allodynia" is:
a. Pain caused by stimuli that are usually not painful
b. The 'burning' sensation of causalgia
c. Red flare with nerve damage
d. Due to reflex sympathetic dystrophy

569. Acute pain:
a. Is usually disproportionate to the injury sustained
b. Is usually self-limiting
c. Cannot affect distant organ systems
d. Is uninfluenced by a patients emotions

570. Nociceptors:
a. Have a fixed threshold for activation
b. Are C fibers; they are myelinated fibers
c. Are encapsulated free nerve endings
d. Capable of encoding stimulus intensity within the noxious range

571. Following is not the side effect of long-term use of strong opioids:
a. Tolerance
b. Addiction
c. Opioid induced hypoalgesia
d. Dependence

572. 40/M, with a history of oral morphine of 200 mg/day, pregabalin 75 mg bd, paractemol of 650 mg BD, posted for laparoscopic pelvic exenteration. Intraoperatively patient received total morphine of 70 mg, paractemol 1 gm, diclofenac 50 mg, and dexmedetomidine infusion of 1 mcg/kg loading followed by 1 mcg/kg/hr maintenance. Intraoperative temperature was maintained to 36 degree. The surgery was uneventful. After reversal of muscle relaxant, anesthetist observed tachycardia to 140 to 150/min, hypotension of 90/50, sweating and pupils were dilated. The drains were normal. The RR is 30 with a good tidal volume. TOF is 95%. What is the likely first step of treatment?
a. Ask the surgeon to convert it to open surgery
b. Give extra reversal agent
c. Extubate
d. IV Morphine/ IV Fentanyl in aliquots titrating the analgesic to keep the respiratory rate between 20 to 25

573. An 18-year-old male, ASA 1, posted for right elbow surgery following trauma, underwent ultrasound guided interscalene block with 20 mL of 0.3% bupivacaine. 20 minutes after the block, just before incision, patient complained of difficulty in opening the eyes. Anesthetist observed right side: small pupils, very slow dilation of pupil to light, drooping of the upper lid, sunken appearance of the eye.

Patient did not complain of any breathing difficulty. Vitals were stable. What will be your next step?
a. Surgery should get postponed
b. Urgent neurology opinion should be taken
c. Proceed with surgery. Patient should be counselled and observed
d. Patient should undergo general anesthesia immediately

574. What is *true* regarding persistent phrenic nerve palsy after interscalene block?
a. It is a rare entity
b. Can be because of triple crush mechanism
c. Double crush syndrome contributes to temporary phrenic nerve palsy
d. Strategies to reduce the risk of the temporary phrenic nerve palsy will also reduce the risk of the permanent phrenic nerve palsy

575. Strategies for reducing phrenic nerve palsy and its clinical impact while ensuring adequate analgesia for shoulder surgery is:
a. Targeting only suprascapular nerve as an alternative to brachial plexus block
b. Limiting the volume of local anesthetic agent to 20 to 25 mL with 0.5% bupivacaine with conventional technique
c. Injection of LA agent 4 mm medial to brachial plexus nerve sheaths
d. Injection of LA agent at superior trunk

576. Following is NOT the nerve block for cleft palate surgery:
a. Infraorbital nerve block
b. Greater palatine nerve block
c. Lesser palatine nerve block
d. Nasopalatine nerve block

577. Which of the following is a *correct* pathway of labor pain?
a. Visceral pain is transmitted by fine, myelinated rapidly transmitting 'A delta' fibers
b. Somatic pain is transmitted by small unmyelinated 'C' fibers
c. The pain of early labor is referred to T10-T12 dermatomes such that pain is felt in the lower abdomen, sacrum and back
d. Somatic pain is from the cutaneous branches of the ilioinguinal and genitofemoral nerves that carry afferent fibers to L1 and L2, only

578. The best choice of maintenance of labor analgesia with minimal complications is:
a. Continuous epidural analgesia with 0.25% bupivacaine @ 10 mL/hr
b. Patient controlled epidural analgesia with a background infusion of 8 mL/hr of 0.1% bupivacaine + Fentanyl 2 mcg/mL with a top ups of 2 mL of 0.1% bupivacaine
c. TENS and entonox combination
d. Continuous spinal analgesia

579. The best approach for sub-Tenon injection of LA in ophthalmic surgery is:
a. Inferonasal
b. Superonasal
c. Lateral canthus
d. Medial canthus

580. A 74-year-old male, with history of recent stroke and MI on medical management had a upper limb fracture due to a fall. He is planned for open reduction and K-wiring of elbow. OT anesthesiologist has an ultrasound image of a regional block that he has planned. See the image and find out his plan.

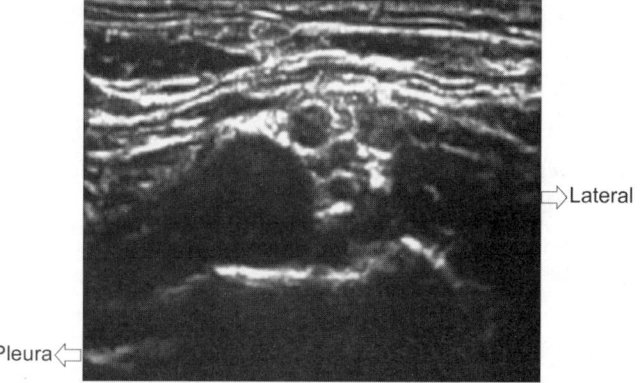

a. Supraclavicular brachial plexus block
b. Infraclavicular brachial plexus block
c. Axillary nerve block
d. Interscalene block

581. A 32-year-old female with h/o CRF and idiopathic pulmonary hypertension posted for plating of a distal end radius fracture. The junior anesthesiologist planned a regional block and missed to block the nerve marked with arrow. Which area of the forearm will be spared, if he has missed to block the nerve that is marked?
a. Posterolateral forearm
b. Anterolateral forearm
c. Anteromedial forearm
d. Posteromedial forearm

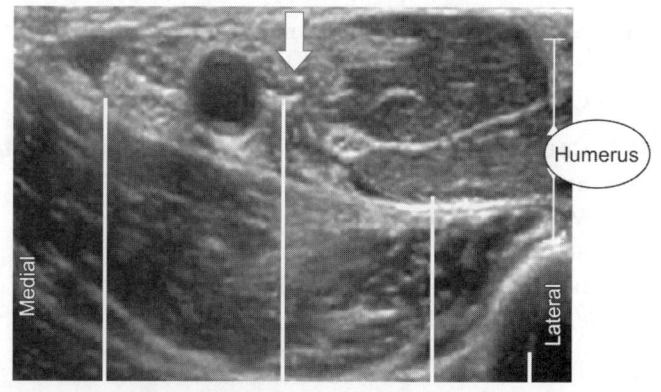

582. A 28-year-old female, with no comorbiditiesis posted for emergency LSCS in view of fetal distress. She is well hydrated. The treating anesthesiologist decides to give spinal anesthesia with 2 mL of 0.5% heavy bupivacaine + Fentanyl 25 mcg. Which of the following is the best option for hemodynamic management of this patient?
   a. Wait for preloading of 250 mL to 500 mL of fluid before giving spinal anesthesia
   b. Co loading of 250 mL of fluid during spinal anesthesia
   c. Treating hypotension with aliquots of ephedrine or phenylephrine
   d. Co-loading of fluid during spinal anesthesia along with aliquots of ephedrine or phenylephrine if required

583. As per practice guideline of obstetric anesthesia, following needle is recommended for spinal anesthesia to avoid PDPH:
   a. Pencil point needle
   b. Cutting needle
   c. 23G needle
   d. 25 G needle

584. A 22-year-old female, underwent emergency open cholecystectomy under general anesthesia at 33 weeks of gestation during her pregnancy. Immediate postoperatively her pain scores were 8/10. What is the best modality of analgesic treatment?
   a. Only Paracetamol (PCM)
   b. PCM + weak opioid
   c. PCM + diclofenac + weak opioid
   d. PCM + diclofenac

585. A 67 year-old male, K/C/O COPD since 10 years, on oral warfarin for chronic atrial fibrillation, is posted for gastrectomy. Patient is also on chronic opioid treatment for gastric cancer-related pain. INR on the day of surgery is 1.6, and WBC 5000. The best and safe analgesic modality will be in case of availability of ultrasound is:
   a. Subcostal TAP block with catheter with post op IV Patient control Analgesia
   b. Lateral TAP block with catheter with post op IV Patient control Analgesia
   c. Posterior TAP block with catheter with post op IV Patient control Analgesia
   d. Epidural analgesia

586. A maxillary nerve block in pterygopalatine fossa blocks following region:
   a. Upper molars
   b. soft palate
   c. Anterior 2/3rd tongue
   d. Ramus of mandible

587. Which of the following steps is not a part of rapid sequence spinal technique?
   a. No touch spinal technique
   b. Limiting the spinal attempts
   c. Use of low dose opioid
   d. Start of surgery before full establishment of the spinal block

588. In pediatric ultrasound guided caudal block, frog eye sign indicates:
   a. Sacral cornua
   b. Sacrococcygeal ligament
   c. Sacral hiatus
   d. Dural sac

589. Which statement is *true* regarding paracetamol?
   a. It is fully absorbed from the stomach
   b. It is an aniline derivative
   c. It is converted to phenacetin
   d. Rate of oral absorption doesn't depends on gastric emptying

590. Cranial nerve most commonly involved after dural puncture:
   a. Abducens   b. Trochlear
   c. Glossophyaryngeal   d. Occulomotor

591. Buprenorphine:
   a. Is a phenanthrene derivative
   b. Has a respiratory depressant action easily antagonised by naloxone
   c. Has high oral bioavailability
   d. May cause withdrawal symptoms in morphine addicts

592. The adverse effects of NSAIDs on the kidney:
   a. Are reversible in normal kidneys
   b. Are not dose related
   c. Can exacerbate effect of loop diuretics
   d. May cause hypokalemia

593. Which of the following is a criterion for the definition of post-surgical chronic pain?
   a. Continuum of acute postoperative pain without an asymptomatic period
   b. Nerve trauma must have been identified intra-operatively
   c. Clinical discomfort for more than 1 month duration
   d. The possibility that the pain is from a preexisting condition has been excluded

594. 54-year/Male, case of carcinoma tongue with complete ankyloglossia is planned for awake tracheal intubation. Patient was given a topical spray with 10% lignocaine. During fibreoptic intubation which of the following reflex is most likely to be blocked?
   a. Cough reflex   b. Gag reflex
   c. Glottic closure reflex   d. Bezold jarisch

595. The simplest scale with accurate clinical to monitor opioid induced sedation is:
   a. Inova Health System Sedation Scale (ISS)
   b. Richmond Agitation and Sedation Scale (RASS)
   c. Pasero Opioid-induced Sedation Scale (POSS)
   d. Glasgow Coma Sedation Scale (GCS)

596. Which of the following is a exclusively a sensory block for knee surgery?
   a. Femoral nerve block
   b. Fascia iliaca block
   c. Adductor canal block
   d. Obturator nerve block

597. Which of the following nerve block is known as "spinal of brachial plexus"?
   a. Interscalene nerve block
   b. Supraclavicular nerve block
   c. Infraclavicular nerve block
   d. Axillary nerve block

598. An ankle block was planned for right foot melanoma excision in 88-year-old male with a H/o of COPD, grade 2 pulmonary hypertension, IHD on medical management with baseline blood pressure as 100/60 and SPO_2 of 94%. After performing the block, majority of plantar surface of the foot, toes, heel was spared. Which nerve block needs to be repeated?
   a. Deep peroneal nerve
   b. Sural nerve
   c. Posterior tibial nerve
   d. Saphenous nerve

599. Which of the following drug has highest oil gas partition coefficient and also highly protein bound?
   a. Lignocaine
   b. Prilocaine
   c. Bupivacaine
   d. Ropivacaine

600. What is the minimum percentage of predicted postoperative FEV_1 below which there is an increased risk of postoperative complications following lobectomy pneumonectomy surgeries?
   a. Lesser than 40%
   b. Lesser than 60%
   c. Lesser than 30%
   d. Lesser than 50%

601. Which one of following elements is included in the three legged stool of preoperative thoracotomy respiratory assessment?
   a. Calculation of dead space
   b. Breath holding time test
   c. Test of response to bronchodilators
   d. Testing for lung parenchymal function – DLCO

602. The circulatory adaptations to cardiac tamponade are:
   a. Decrease PCWP and increase in LV, RV, and RA pressures
   b. Increase PCWP and decrease in LV, RV, and RA pressures
   c. Decrease in PCWP, LV, RV, and RA pressures
   d. Increase in PCWP, LV, RV, and RA pressures

603. Protamine reaction with features of anaphylactoid reactions is:
   a. Type I
   b. Type IV
   c. Type II
   d. Type III

604. Which of the following is *true* about epinephrine?
   a. It has no beta receptor activity
   b. A dose of >10 ug/min activates beta receptors and increases heart rate and contractility
   c. Higher doses of epinephrine cause reflex bradycardia due to increase in blood pressure
   d. It is a potent renal vasodilator

605. Desensitization block occurs when:
   a. The receptor is in a resting state
   b. The binding of the agonist to the receptor does not cause opening of the channel
   c. The receptor does not bind to the agonist
   d. The receptor binds to the antagonist

606. The following is *true* about methaemoglobinaemia
   a. Increased binding of Hb molecule to oxygen
   b. The cyanosis is responsive to supplemental oxygen
   c. Important causes are dapsone and benzocaine in susceptible patients
   d. Oxygen delivery remains normal

607. The quantity of CO_2 in the arterial and mixed venous blood is:
   a. 21.5 and 23.3 mmol/Lit of blood respectively
   b. 35 and 19 mmol/Lit of blood respectively
   c. 26 and 24.5 mmol/Lit of blood respectively
   d. 15 and 45 mmol/Lit of blood respectively

608. The human brain receives ___% of the cardiac output
   a. 5–10%
   b. 20–30%
   c. 12–15%
   d. 2–3%

609. Regarding the effect of anesthetic agents on cerebral metabolic rate (CMR) which of these will NOT suppress the EEG activity?
   a. Barbiturates
   b. Propofol
   c. Inhalational agents
   d. Nitrous oxide

610. Which one of the following equations best describes the relation between alveolar and minute ventilation?
 (V_E = minute ventilation, V_D = dead space, V_A = alveolar ventilation)
 a. $V_E = V_A + fx\, V_D$
 b. $V_E = V_A - fx\, V_D$
 c. $V_E = V_A - fxV_D$
 d. $V_E = V_A/fx\, V_D$

611. Regarding pressure volume curves of the lung, which of the following is *true*?
 a. In fibrosis, there is an increase in the slope of the curve
 b. In bronchitis, there is an upward shift of the curve
 c. In emphysema, there is flattening of the curve
 d. In asthma, the curve indicates increase in compliance

612. Which of the following is *true* about deep hypothermic circulatory arrest (DHCA)?
 a. It means reducing the patients body temperature to <10°C
 b. It is used to prevent the heart from ischemic insults
 c. It is primarily used in surgical repair of aorta
 d. The viscosity of blood decreases as the patient cools

613. Risk factor for patients undergoing CABG surgery include?
 a. LVEF 45%
 b. Younger age groups <25 years
 c. No history of previous cardiac surgery
 d. Obesity

614. As per the AHA classification of stages of chronic heart failure, what is Stage C?
 a. Symptomatic heart failure with dyspnea, fatigue and impaired exercise tolerance
 b. End stage heart failure with marked symptoms at rest
 c. Heart failure with valvular dysfunction
 d. Biventricular heart failure

615. The maximum allowable radiation limit for a medical worker in one lifetime is:
 a. 5 rem/year
 b. 1 rem × age
 c. 2 rad/year
 d. 50 rad/year

616. Which of the following is a risk factor for low cardiac output syndrome (LCOS) after cardiopulmonary bypass
 a. Obesity
 b. Previous history of cardiac surgery
 c. Intraoperative hypotension
 d. Reperfusion injury

617. In the RIFLE classification of acute kidney injury, failure is defined as:
 a. Plasma creatinine increase 1.5 times
 b. Urine output <0.5 mL/kg/hr for 12 hours
 c. Complete loss of kidney function >4 weeks
 d. Urine output <0.3 mL/kg/hr for 24 hours

618. Which of the following physiological change occurs with aortic cross clamping?
 a. Increased blood pressure above the clamp
 b. Increased total body oxygen consumption
 c. Decreased mixed venous oxygen saturation
 d. Respiratory acidosis

619. Which of the following is *true* about aortic unclamping?
 a. Increased myocardial contractility
 b. Metabolic alkalosis
 c. Decreased venous return
 d. Increased arterial blood pressure

620. Most sensitive method for detecting an intraoperative venous air embolism (VAE) is:
 a. Esophageal stethoscope
 b. Trans-esophageal echo
 c. Pulmonary artery pressure
 d. Capnograph ($EtCO_2$)

621. Which of the following is a part metabolic syndrome?
 a. Abdominal obesity
 b. IHD
 c. High HDL cholesterol
 d. High heart rate

622. Which of the following is *true* about obstructive sleep apnea (OSA)?
 a. Apnea should last at least 20 seconds
 b. At least 10 or more such episodes per hour of sleep
 c. 70% cessation of airflow
 d. Accompanied by at least 4% decrease in saturation

623. Which one of these drugs is completely dependent on the kidney for its excretion?
 a. Barbiturates   b. Digoxin
 c. Neostigmine   d. Hydralazine

624. Of the following, which is the commonest cause of immediate postoperative jaundice?
 a. Blood transfusion
 b. Total parenteral nutrition (TPN)
 c. Post-intestinal bypass
 d. Bile duct stricture

625. Which of the following is *true* about extended donor criteria for kidney?
 a. Donors >30 years of age
 b. Pre-terminal serum creatinine <1 mg/dL

c. Age >60 years
d. Death caused by cancer of non-renal origin

626. The trace element catalyzing hemoglobin synthesis is:
a. Manganese
b. Magnesium
c. Copper
d. Selenium

627. Which of the following is *true* about the determination of brain death?
a. The patient should be sedated but not paralyzed
b. Systolic blood pressure >130 mm Hg
c. Core temperature >36°C
d. Hypercarbia

628. Method of ancillary testing for determination of brain death does not include which one of the following?
a. Bispectral index monitoring (BIS)
b. EEG
c. Transcranial doppler
d. Cerebral scinitgraphy

629. Which one of the following is *true* about the physiological changes of pregnancy?
a. Plasma volume increases 45-55%
b. Increase in central venous pressure
c. Increase in platelet count by 10%
d. Erythrocytes decrease by 10%

630. Which of the following is *true* about aorto-caval compression syndrome?
a. There is an increase in cardiac output and stroke volume by 10%
b. Decrease in sympathetic tone
c. It is also known as supine hypotension syndrome
d. Anesthesia reduces its occurrence

631. What is *true* about maternal laparoscopy?
a. Low tidal volume ventilation should be encouraged
b. Laparoscopic surgeries should be performed after second trimester
c. End tidal CO_2 and arterial CO_2 gradient should be <5 mm Hg
d. Gasless techniques should be avoided

632. Which of the following is *true* about anesthesia for fetal surgery?
a. Maternal FiO_2 should be >80%
b. $EtCO_2$ should be maintained in higher normal range (40-45 mm Hg)
c. At least 6 minutes of preoxygenation should be done
d. Rapid sequence induction should be done

633. Which one of the following is not a major criterion for detection of fat embolism?
a. Anemia
b. Petechial rash
c. Cerebral involvement
d. Respiratory insufficiency

634. Which of the following is NOT a risk factor for post-operative delirium?
a. Diabetes
b. Decreased oral intake
c. Sleep deprivation
d. Immobility

635. Which of the following is *true* about the consequences of aggressive volume replacement in early resuscitation?
a. Increased clotting factor concentration
b. Increased blood viscosity
c. Increased hematocrit
d. Electrolyte imbalance

636. Which of the following is NOT a goal for early resuscitation?
a. Systolic blood pressure >120 mm Hg
b. Hematocrit 25-30%
c. Platelet count >50,000/hpf
d. Core temperature >35°C

637. Which of the following is NOT *true* regarding anesthesia for limb surgery following trauma?
a. Regional anesthesia increases the risk of DVT
b. General anesthesia can make hemodynamic management more complex
c. Need for sedation is common with regional anesthesia
d. Better pulmonary toileting is not possible with regional anesthesia

638. Which of the following is NOT a risk factor for development of compartment syndrome?
a. Burns
b. Snakebite
c. Exploratory laparotomy surgeries
d. Intraosseous fluid replacement in children

639. Which is NOT *true* about airway fire prevention?
a. Keep FiO_2 at least 50%
b. N_2O should be avoided
c. Endotracheal tube cuff should be filled with saline
d. Incase of a fire, field should be flooded with saline

640. Which of the following is NOT *true* regarding oculocardiac reflex?
a. It is also called Aschner Dagnini reflex
b. Bradycardia

c. If suspected, the surgeon should be asked to stop the surgical manipulations
d. Efferent limb is via the trigeminal nerve

641. Which of the following is *true* about lasers?
    a. Class I lasers are safe under all conditions
    b. Class IIIb lasers are dangerous if viewed for >2 minutes
    c. Class IIIa lasers are safe up to 1000 seconds of continual viewing
    d. Class IV lasers are safe because of blink reflex

642. Which of the following is *true* about modified Aldrete score?
    a. Score <9 requires ICU admission
    b. Score of at least 10 is required to discharge from recovery
    c. Patients moving all four limbs voluntarily are given 2 points
    d. Blood pressure 20–49% of baseline is given 2 points

643. A 35-year-old patient has severe laryngospasm after extubation of the trachea following general anesthesia. Administration of 100% oxygen using continuous positive airway pressure does not improve symptoms. SpO$_2$ is 75%. Which of the following is the most appropriate immediate management?
    a. Laryngeal mask airway
    b. Racemic epinephrine
    c. Succinylcholine
    d. Cricothyroidotomy

644. Following pneumonectomy, a paralyzed patient being mechanically ventilated has the following arterial blood gas values: PaO$_2$ 81 mm Hg, PaCO$_2$ 55 mm Hg, pH 7.29. SvO$_2$ is 45%. The most likely explanation for this ScvO$_2$ is:
    a. Decreased red cell mass
    b. High cardiac output
    c. Hypothermia
    d. Ventilation perfusion mismatch

645. A morbidly obese patient is scheduled for gastric stapling during general anesthesia. Following preoxygenation and induction, the oxygen saturation decreases after 45 seconds of laryngoscopy and attempted intubation. The rapid onset of arterial desaturation is most likely due to:
    a. Aspiration during induction
    b. Decreased functional residual capacity
    c. Increased cardiac output
    d. Increased ventilatory dead space

646. A patient has hoarseness after undergoing surgery involving the aortic arch. The most likely cause is an injury to which of the following nerves?
    a. Glossopharyngeal
    b. Left recurrent laryngeal
    c. Right recurrent laryngeal
    d. Left superior laryngeal

647. Which of the following is not a feature of ARDS?
    a. No evidence of cardiac failure
    b. Bilateral diffuse infiltrates on chest X-ray
    c. Protein low fluid in alveolar space
    d. Refractory hypoxia

648. Which one of the following patients is the most appropriate candidate for noninvasive positive pressure ventilation?
    a. 35-year-old immunosuppressed female with lung infiltrates and respiratory failure
    b. 67-year-old male POD 6 esophagectomy with witnessed aspiration
    c. 45-year-old female with advanced cirrhosis and hepatopulmonary syndrome
    d. 35-year-old female with septic shock and arterial desaturation

649. A 40-year-old patient with history of metastatic carcinoma of breast presents from oncology ward to ICU. She complains of shortness of breath and tachypnea. Her blood pressure is 130/80 mmHg and SpO$_2$ is 96% on 4 liter of oxygen/minute, using nasal cannula. An X-ray chest is shown. What is the most probable cause of her clinical presentation?
    a. Malignant pleural effusion
    b. Pulmonary embolism
    c. Pneumonia
    d. Pneumothorax

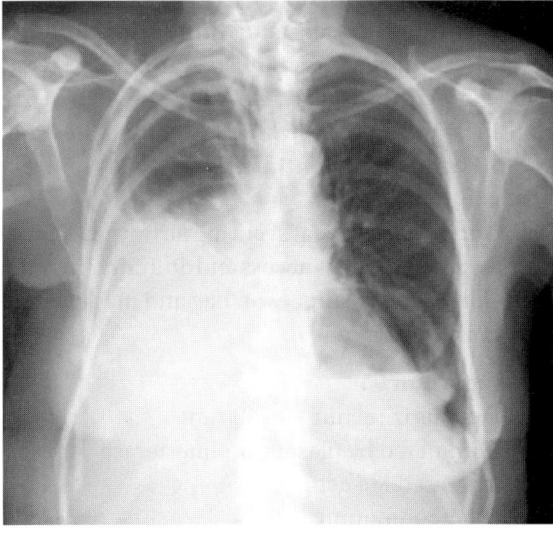

650. Which of the following valves prevents transfilling between compressed gas cylinders?
    a. Fail-safe valve
    b. Pop-off valve

c. Adjustable pressure-limiting valve
d. Check valve

651. Which of the following pulmonary function tests is least dependent on patient effort?
    a. Forced expiratory volume in 1 second (FEV1)
    b. Forced vital capacity (FVC)
    c. FEF 25–75%
    d. Maximum voluntary ventilation (MVV)

652. Hepatocellular integrity of tissue is assessed by which of the following tests?
    a. Bilirubin
    b. Gamma glutamyl transferase
    c. Albumin
    d. Aspartate amino transferase and alanine amino transferase

653. A 32-year-old male patient of RTA with fracture shaft femur is posted for fixation. During shifting to the OR table, the patient suddenly became drowsy and disoriented. He became hypotensive (BP- 70/30 mmHg) and desaturated (SpO$_2$: 60%). What is the most likely cause?
    a. Pulse oximeter was not attached properly
    b. Deranged serum sodium
    c. Fat embolism
    d. Massive blood loss

654. A victim of RTA with head injury opens eyes to pain, keeps mumbling, and withdraws his hand on painful stimulus. What is his Glasgow Coma Score?
    a. 3
    b. 7
    c. 8
    d. 9

655. While administering GA for an elective surgery in a child, 3 attempts at intubation failed. Mask ventilation was possible, so 2 attempts at securing airway with different supraglottic airway devices (SGAD) were made, which also failed. Rescue mask ventilation was continued. What is the next best step?
    a. Another attempt at securing airway with SGAD
    b. Take front of neck access and do a cricothyroidotomy
    c. Continue the surgery on bag and mask ventilation
    d. Wake the patient up

656. Mivacurium is:
    a. Depolarizing muscle relaxant
    b. Eliminated by plasma cholinesterase
    c. Intermediate acting
    d. Ester compound

657. Which of the following drugs is contraindicated in porphyria?
    a. Ketamine
    b. Propofol
    c. Thiopentone
    d. Fentanyl

658. Which local anesthetic agent has an inherent vasoconstrictor activity:
    a. Prilocaine
    b. Cocaine
    c. EMLA
    d. Lignocaine

659. A 45-year-old female has undergone laparoscopic cholecystectomy. Which of the following blocks will provide the best postoperative analgesia?
    a. Transversalis fascia plane block
    b. Bilateral rectus sheath block
    c. Quadratus lumborum block
    d. Rectus sheath block and subcostal transversus abdominis plane block

660. The driving force for the piston ventilators on the anesthesia workstation is provided by:
    a. Nitrous oxide
    b. Compressed oxygen
    c. Electricity
    d. Electricity and air

661. A 2-year-old child with Treacher's collin syndrome is posted for cleft palate repair surgery. Securing airway with endotracheal tube is best accomplished by:
    a. Awake nasal intubation with topical anesthesia
    b. Intravenous induction with succinylcoline and then securing the airway
    c. Administering Inhalational agent sevoflurane and spontaneous ventilation
    d. Nasal intubation after IM ketamine administration

662. Which of the following is the most likely effect of administration of magnesium sulfate in a patient with preeclampsia?
    a. Decreased motor end-plate sensitivity to acetylcholine
    b. Decreased uteroplacental blood flow
    c. Increased systemic vascular resistance
    d. Inhibits acetylcholinesterase

663. MAC value of Xenon is:
    a. 84%
    b. 71%
    c. 62%
    d. 45%

664. A 28-year-old female underwent cesarean section under spinal anesthesia, two days later she is afebrile but has severe occipital pain that is aggravated by sitting or standing and relieved by lying flat. Associated findings with it would likely include:
    a. Bradycardia
    b. Difficulty swallowing
    c. Diplopia
    d. Horner's syndrome

665. Steal induction is:
    a. The child taken away from the mother to the operating room by showing cartoons on the mobile phone
    b. Child is brought to operating room using force and physical restraint
    c. Child comes to the operating room already asleep undergoing anesthesia induction without being awakened
    d. Steal induction is done only with ketamine

666. Which of the following drugs is preferred for treatment of hyperthyroidism in pregnant women?
    a. Propylthiouracil
    b. Carbimazole
    c. Methimazole
    d. Iodine

667. A 67-year-old man undergoes a perineal procedure under spinal anesthesia in the lithotomy position with extreme flexion of the thigh at the hip. No sedatives are used, and the surgery is uneventful. 24 hours later, the patient cannot flex his left knee. Which of the following is the most likely cause?
    a. Epidural hematoma
    b. L5 nerve root injury
    c. Peroneal nerve injury
    d. Sciatic nerve injury

668. Inhalational induction is faster in infants than adults because:
    a. Infants have low minute ventilation-to-FRC ratio
    b. Infants have lower alveolar ventilation and lower FRC compared to adults
    c. Infants have higher alveolar ventilation and higher FRC compared to adults
    d. Infants have higher minute ventilation-to-FRC ratio

669. At equipotent doses, which of the following opioids is most likely to migrate cephalad in cerebrospinal fluid?
    a. Fentanyl
    b. Meperidine
    c. Morphine
    d. Sufentanil

670. In patients with pregnancy-induced hypertension, magnesium sulphate is most likely to:
    a. Increase maternal heart rate
    b. Decrease sensitivity to relaxants
    c. Decrease succinylcholine-induced fasciculations
    d. Prevent hypokalemia

671. The four E-type oxygen cylinders are there on an anesthesia machine and have pressure readings of 1100 psig each. At an oxygen flow of 5 L/min, there will be sufficient oxygen for approximately:
    a. 3 hours
    b. 4 hours
    c. 5 hours
    d. 1 hour

672. As compared with atracurium, Cis-atracurium
    a. Is less hemodynamically stable
    b. Is associated with less/almost nil histamine release
    c. Has slower neuromuscular blocking activity
    d. Is less potent

673. Which one of the following increases cerebral blood flow while decreasing cerebral metabolic rate?
    a. Etomidate
    b. Fentanyl
    c. Desflurane
    d. Isoflurane

674. Which of the following is a strong ion?
    a. PO_4
    b. Albumin
    c. Cl^-
    d. HCO_3^-

675. Von Willebrand factor binds to which of the following platelet glycoprotein receptors?
    a. GP IV
    b. GP Ib-IX
    c. GP IIb-IIIa
    d. GP Ia-IIa

676. Which of the following is a prodrug?
    a. Parecoxib
    b. Celecoxib
    c. Valdecoxib
    d. Lumiracoxib

677. Which of the following is metabolized by CYP2D6?
    a. Oxycodone
    b. Morphine
    c. Buprenorphine
    d. Codeine

678. What is the optimal range for damping coefficient of arterial blood pressure transducer system?
    a. 0.41–0.83
    b. 0.32–0.54
    c. 0.64 and 0.77
    d. 1.2–1.1

679. Which of the following is *true* about ketamine?
    a. It is a competitive antagonist at the NMDA receptor
    b. R (–) isomer has lesser incidence of emergence phenomena
    c. Has high hepatic extraction ratio
    d. Protein binding is 99%

680. Which of the following drugs is least likely to affect the QT interval?
    a. Ondansetron
    b. Droperidol
    c. Granisetron
    d. Palonosetron

681. Which of the following does not cross the blood brain barrier?
    a. Domperidone
    b. Ondansetron
    c. Metoclopramide
    d. Scopolamine

682. What is the mechanism of propofol infusion syndrome?
    a. Hyperchloremic metabolic acidosis
    b. Cytotoxic hypoxia
    c. Sepsis
    d. Renal failure

683. Which of the following drugs decreases lower esophageal sphincter tone?
    a. Neostigmine
    b. Progesterone
    c. Metoclopramide
    d. Domperidone

684. Which of the following delays gastric emptying?
    a. Secretin
    b. Neostigmine
    c. Gastrin
    d. Alkalosis

685. What is the threshold of change in serum osmolality for release of ADH from posterior pituitary?
    a. 10%
    b. 5%
    c. 1%
    d. 20%

686. In the Bezold–Jarisch reflex, a decrease in left ventricular volume causes which of the following?
    a. Tachycardia
    b. Bradycardia
    c. Hypotension
    d. Hypertension

687. The most common cause of inhibition of pyruvate dehydrogenase is:
    a. Cardiogenic shock
    b. Septic shock
    c. Obstructive shock
    d. Anaphylactic shock

688. Which ONE of the following is an octapeptide?
    a. Angiotensin II
    b. Angiotensinogen
    c. Angiotensin I
    d. Angiotensin III

689. At the end of Cori's cycle, where lactate is converted to glucose, there is:
    a. Net gain of 6 ATPs
    b. Net loss of 6 ATPs
    c. Net gain of 4 ATPs
    d. Net loss of 4 ATPs

690. The cardiovascular consequences of metabolic acidosis include all of the following, *except:*
    a. Increased heart rate and contractility at pH >7.2
    b. Decreased contractility at pH <7.1
    c. Increased cardiac responsiveness to catecholamines
    d. Decreased fibrillation threshold

691. Delayed sequence intubation (DSI), which is now commonly used in ED and ICU consists of which one of the following?
    a. Temporal separation of injection of induction agent and muscle relaxant
    b. Simultaneous administration of induction agent and muscle relaxant using 2 IV catheters
    c. Injection of induction agent followed immediately by muscle relaxant
    d. Injection of a benzodiazepine and fentanyl and no muscle relaxant

692. In the new concept of physiologically difficult airway in the critically ill, the difficulty is due to all of the following, *except:*
    a. Hypoxemia
    b. Hypotension
    c. Severe metabolic acidosis
    d. Left ventricular failure

693. Which of the following is the Gold Standard for confirming the tracheal placement of the endotracheal tube?
    a. Ultrasonography of the airway
    b. Five point auscultation
    c. Colorimetric method
    d. Capnography

694. On performing direct laryngoscopy, only the very posterior part of vocal cords is visible, this indicates:
    a. Cormack Lehane Grade I view
    b. Cormack Lehane Grade Ia view
    c. Cormack Lehane Grade III view
    d. Cormack Lehane Grade IIb view

695. Context-sensitive half-life or context-sensitive half-time is defined as:
    a. The time taken for blood plasma concentration of a drug to decline by 48% after the bolus dose has been injected
    b. The time taken for blood plasma concentration of a drug to decline by 50% after the infusion has been stopped
    c. The time taken for blood plasma concentration of a drug to decline by 50% after a 48 hr mandatory infusion has been stopped
    d. The time taken for blood plasma concentration of a drug to decline by 55% after the infusion has been stopped

696. The statement "Phenytoin follows nonlinear kinetics at therapeutic concentrations," means:
    a. Concentration of phenytoin decreases in an unpredictable manner
    b. Concentration of phenytoin decreases depending on the plasma concentration of the drug
    c. Concentration of phenytoin decreases depending on the liver function of the patient
    d. Concentration of phenytoin decreases in a predictable manner

697. A 22-year-old boy presented to the emergency department after a vehicular accident. On examination he is confused, his pulse rate is 128/min, blood pressure is 88/68 mmHg and his urine output for the last hour has been 10 mL. According to the ATLS classification, he is in which class of hemorrhagic shock?
    a. Class I
    b. Class II
    c. Class III
    d. Class IV

698. Which overdose may not benefit from a bicarbonate infusion?
    a. Cyclic antidepressant overdose
    b. Salicylate overdose
    c. Methanol ingestion
    d. Digoxin overdose

699. Which of the following is *true* regarding Doppler ultrasound?
    a. Uses same transducer crystals to transmit and receive ultrasound
    b. Can be used to measure systemic blood pressure
    c. Measurements are unaffected by movement
    d. Red indicates arterial blood flow and blue indicates venous blood flow

700. Which of the following is not Gram Positive Bacteria?
    a. *Staphylococcus aureus*
    b. *Enterococcus faecalis*
    c. *Enterobacter aerogenes*
    d. *Listeria monocytogene*

ANSWERS

1. **(b). 50 mL/100 g/min**
   The global CBF in adults is about 50 mL/100 g/min. Children have a higher CBF, approximately 95 mL/100 g/min. In contrast, infants have a slightly lower CBF around 40 mL/100 mg/min.

2. **(b). 65**
   Cerebral perfusion pressure is derived by the formulae: MAP – ICP or CVP, whichever is higher.
   So in our case, CVP is higher and that is why: CPP: 80–15 : 65 mm Hg.

3. **(c). Ketamine**
   All intravenous induction agents, *except* Ketamine, are cerebral vasoconstrictors and cause dose-dependent decreases in cerebral metabolic rate and CBF. Ketamine is a cerebral vasodilator and thus increases the CBF.

4. **(a). Rocuronium**
   Muscle relaxants have no effect on SSEPs. All inhalational volatile anesthetics, Propofol and Narcotics, in a dose-dependent manner, decrease the amplitude and increase latency of the SSEPs.

5. **(d). Brainstem auditory-evoked potentials (BAEP)**
   BAEP is used to test the auditory pathways following stimulation of the cochlear nerve. Early latency BAEP are resistant to the anesthetic effects. Use of drill during surgeries interferes with the auditory stimuli and waveforms get distorted. Damage to the cochlear vessel (or vasospasm) abolishes all the waveforms and thus not helpful in brainstem monitoring.

6. **(d). Mean arterial pressure targets should be set to >90 mm Hg following clipping of the aneurysm**
   The peak incidence of vasospasm occurs between days 5 and 10. The magnesium for aneurysmal subarachnoid hemorrhage (MASH) 2 trial showed no benefit to magnesium supplementation, and 'triple H' therapy is now suggested to be potentially harmful, *except* the Hypertension part. MAP targets aim to restore CPP, with a target of >60 mm Hg until the aneurysm is clipped (to limit the risk of further bleeding) and a target of >90 mm Hg following clipping.

7. **(c). Absent cough reflex response to bronchial stimulation by a suction catheter placed down the trachea to the carina**
   The pupils are fixed and do not respond to sharp changes in light intensity and are dilated. Measurement of visual evoked responses alone is not confirmatory of brainstem death, it is one of the ancillary test to help support diagnosis along with other tests like EEG, brainstem auditory evoked potentials. Spinal reflexes to a sternal rub can still occur and do not signify brainstem function.

8. **(b). Ehlers-Danlos syndrome**
   Risk factors for aneurysmal subarachnoid hemorrhage (SAH) include hypertension, smoking, alcohol abuse, female sex, a strong family history and certain genetic syndromes, such as autosomal dominant polycystic kidney disease and collagen disorders such as Type IV Ehlers-Danlos syndrome.

9. **(a). There is progressive bradycardia and hypotension due to the developing spinal shock**
   In high cervical cord lesions, the interruption of sympathetic outflow can lead to the development of neurogenic shock, with resultant bradycardia and hypotension. This is often confused with spinal shock, which actually refers to the absence of reflexes below the level of the lesion caused by a transient 'concussion' of the cord.

10. **(d). When the amplitude of P2 exceeds P1 this is suggestive of reduced brain compliance**
    Lundberg A waves are always pathological and indicate steep rise in ICP to about 50 mm Hg or more and persist for 5–20 mins and are therefore also called as plateau waves. P1 wave, also called as percussion wave, corresponds to choroid plexus pulsations and P2 wave, also called as dicrotic wave, corresponds to closure of aortic valve. In normal patients, the amplitude of P1 exceeds P2.

11. **(a). Peripherally injected drugs should be flushed with at least 20 mL of fluid followed by arm raise**
    Drug dosages are equivalent when administered via the intravenous and intraosseous routes. The humerus and tibia have equal flow rates for fluids. Tracheal administration leads to variable plasma concentrations of drugs and with the advent of newer devices making intraosseous access easier, tracheal drug administration is no longer recommended.

12. **(c). Steroids**
    Treatment of intracranial hypertension includes hyperventilation to $PaCO_2$ of 25–30 mm Hg, using an osmotic diuretic (mannitol), hypertonic saline, improving CSF drainage by elevating the head by 30 degrees or surgical placement of CSF drain, decompression craniectomy, barbiturates, and corticosteroids. The latter have been mainly used to decrease cerebral edema caused by tumors in the supratentorial region and not routinely recommended as a routine for all cases.

13. **(a). Start CPR, beginning with chest compressions**
    Follow each shock immediately with CPR, beginning with compressions. A shock stuns the heart and abolishes the arrhythmia which led to cardiac arrest. A normal perfusing rhythm will not return immediately and so no point wasting time by doing unnecessary pulse checks.

14. **(b). 30 : 2**
    When there is no advanced airway in place, one should do CPR cycle of 30 compressions and 2 breaths. Once advanced airway is in place, compression should continue continuously at 100–120/min and breaths should be given one every 6 minutes.

15. **(a). Early CPR and early defibrillation**
    BLS ensures that basic life-saving measures are implemented as soon as possible whether or not a healthcare provider is available. Early CPR and early defibrillation improve outcomes for patients with cardiac arrest.
    Rhythm interpretation and advanced airway and drugs form part of the ACLS.

16. **(c). Team members do not question team leaders orders even if doubt exists**
    The team leader should encourage team members to participate in leadership and not simply follow directions blindly. He assigns clear roles and responsibilities to all team members and the team members too should respect each other and provide constructive interventions as required.

17. **(a). Make sure the scene is safe**
    Prior to conducting the BLS, primary, and secondary assessments, make sure that the scene is safe. One can help the victim only if there is no threat to caregiver, we do not want one more victim.

18. **(a). Chest compressions, airway, breathing**
    The BLS sequence for CPR is C-A-B (compressions, airway, breathing). This places emphasis on minimizing delays and interruptions of chest compressions.

19. **(d). Use an immobilization device to stabilize the head**
    In the trauma patient with a suspected neck injury, use jaw thrust without head extension. Maintaining a patent airway and providing ventilation are priorities, so if the jaw thrust is not effective, use a head tilt-chin lift maneuver. Use manual spinal motion restriction rather than immobilization devices as it is safer.

20. **(b). Obtain IV access, attach ECG leads, monitor rhythm, given medications to manage rhythm, give IV/IO fluids if needed**
    Actions performed in the circulation portion of the primary assessment all involve some aspect of assessment or treatment of the cardiovascular system. Airway comes in the breathing portion of the primary assessment.

21. **(d). Disability**
    It mainly involves a quick general neurological assessment which includes assessment of responsiveness, level of consciousness, and pupil reflex. The AVPU acronym helps (Alert, Voice, Painful, Unresponsive).

22. **(a). Atropine, epinephrine, dopamine**
    Atropine is used to increase the heart rate, but repeat doses to be used with caution in second degree type 2 and third degree AV heart block. Epinephrine and dopamine are both used as an alternative to transcutaneous pacing (TCP) as infusions.

23. **(a). 5–20 mcg/kg/min infusion**
    Dopamine infusion is to be started at 5–20 mcg/kg/min and titrated to adequate perfusion and patient response.

24. **(a). 1 mg atropine, may repeat up to a total dose of 3 mg**
    Atropine 1 mg is given IV every 3–5 minutes. The dosage has been revised in the 2020 guidelines from 0.5 to 1 mg.

25. **(a). Unstable atrial fibrillation**
    The treatment for unstable tachyarrhythmia is synchronized cardioversion. Pulseless VT and VF are arrest rhythms and need CPR and defibrillation.

26. **(a). Epinephrine**
    Epinephrine is used in cardiac arrest algorithm as a bolus of 1 mg and in symptomatic bradyarrhythmias an infusion.

27. **(b). Brachial pulse**
    In infants it is difficult to check the carotid pulse due to their short neck. In older children, the femoral pulse can also be used for pulse check.

28. **(d). Adenosine 6 mg**
    Stable tachyarrhythmia are treated with vagal maneuvers followed by adenosine 6 mg. A second dose of adenosine can be given of 12 mg if the first has been ineffective after 3–5 minutes. One should however be cautious while using Adenosine in asthmatics as can cause bronchospasm.

29. **(d). Epinephrine 1 mg IV**
    The only drug to be given in asystole is epinephrine 1 mg IV every 3–5 minutes. The IV route is preferred over the ETT route as more reliable for drug absorption and action.

30. **(d). Amiodarone 300 mg**
    Vasopressin is no longer found to be beneficial and does not have any role in arrest protocol. Lidocaine can

be given as a substitute of epinephrine and not as a following drug to epinephrine. So the next drug in line to be given for refractory pulseless VT is amiodarone 300 mg as IV bolus.

31. **(a). Hypertension**
Clinical signs of venous air embolism include a decrease in end-tidal CO_2, a decrease in arterial oxygen saturation, sudden hypotension, mill wheel murmur, and even sudden circulatory arrest. The severity of symptoms depends on the amount and rate at which air enters the venous system. The adult lethal volume has been reported as 3–4 mL/kg.

32. **(a). Transesophageal echocardiogram (TEE)**
The most sensitive and gold standard intraoperative monitor for detecting venous air embolism is TEE. It can detect 0.02 mL/kg of air as compared to the second best monitor, precordial Doppler sonography, which can detect as little as 0..05 mL/kg of air. Changes in end-tidal respiratory gas concentrations, such as nitrogen and carbon dioxide, and changes in pulmonary artery pressures are less sensitive. Hypotension and mill wheel murmur are late manifestations of venous air embolism.

33. **(c). Level of external auditory meatus**
In a seated/semi-seated patient, the arterial pressure in the brain differs significantly from left ventricular pressure. CPP is determined by setting the transducer to zero at the level of the ear, which approximates to the circle of Willis.

34. **(c). Total volume of CSF is about 150 mL**
CSF is formed by the choroid plexuses of cerebral lateral ventricles and absorbed in arachnoid granulations over cerebral hemispheres. CSF formation involves active secretion of sodium in the choroid plexuses, and not passive diffusion. In adults, normal CSF production is about 20 mL/hour with a total volume of 150 mL.

35. **(a). Hypotension**
The acromegalic patient suffers from general overgrowth of skeletal, soft, and connective tissues resulting in coarse facial features and enlarged hands and feet. Patients may also have a difficult airway because of overgrowth of soft tissues of upper airway, enlargement of tongue and epiglottis, overgrowth of mandible with increased distance from lips to vocal cords, and glottic and subglottic narrowing. These changes may also lead to obstructive sleep apnea. Patients also are prone to hyperglycemia, hypertension, congestive heart failure, increased lung volumes, increased ventilation–perfusion mismatch, peripheral neuropathy, skeletal muscle weakness, osteoarthritis, and osteoporosis.

36. **(d). A GCS of 6 means the patient is in coma**
The GCS is a three-point scale used to describe the level of consciousness in patients with head injury. The highest score is 15 (normal) and the lowest score is 3 (deep coma). The patient is assessed on ability to open eyes, motor responses and vocalization. A patient of GCS 8 (with no eye opening) or less is considered to be in coma.

37. **(a). At the moment of impact**
Primary brain injury describes the injury that happens at the moment of impact or injury.

38. **(a). 50–150 mm Hg**
The brain does not have large stores of glucose or oxygen and is dependent on CBF to deliver these essential substrates. CBF is therefore tightly regulated and kept constant despite changes in the MAP between a range of 50–150 mm Hg. The various mechanism in play are the myogenic and metabolic activity.

39. **(a). The syndrome of inappropriate secretion of antidiuretic hormone (SIADH)**
Hyponatremia is often caused by SIADH and is caused by the kidneys holding on to water due to the action of excess ADH on the renal tubules. The total body sodium is normal but total body water is increased. Sodium is low due to a dilutional effect and water restriction can be used to treat this condition. Diabetes insipidus is caused by lack of secretion of ADH and causes a high urine output and dehydration as the kidneys are unable to concentrate the urine. The sodium will rise (hypernatremia). Diabetes mellitus (raised blood glucose) is common in severely injured patients but is not a cause of hyponatremia. Increased cortisol secretion will occur as part of the stress response to injury but will not cause hyponatremia.

40. **(b). 5%**
Late seizures occur in 5% of patients with closed head injury and 15% of patients with severe head injuries. Seizures can usually be controlled with anticonvulsants.

41. **(b). It produces pain out of all proportion to the injury**
Compartment syndrome is a surgical emergency. Although it is normally associated with a closed fracture, it can result from any blunt trauma and the bone does not need to be fractured. The distal pulses and even sensation may be unimpaired, because the arteries still pump blood, and if the distal nerve does not pass through that compartment it will be unaffected. The patient experiences pain out of all proportion to the injury, and if the muscles are stretched (passive extension), the patient experiences extreme pain. The pressure in the compartment needs to be

released within hours if permanent damage is to be avoided.

42. **(a). Reduction in venous blood volume**
An expanding mass lesion will initially cause reduction in venous blood volume and CSF volume and therefore pressure will remain constant. As the mass lesion increases, it may compress the brain. Arterial volume is maintained until the late stages. At a certain point the mass lesion will overcome the compensatory mechanisms and ICP will start to rise. At this point, small increases in volume will cause large increases in pressure. This can be shown as a pressure–volume curve.

43. **(c). Magnetic resonance imaging (MRI)**
As the patient is unconscious, it can be difficult to 'clear' the cervical spine. Plain X-rays will not be adequate and flexion and extension views carry an unquantified risk of causing further damage. The patient should certainly not be left on a spine board any longer than absolutely necessary because of the risk of causing bed sores. An MRI would be the safest and most reliable way of ruling out an unstable spine injury.

44. **(d). The cervicothoracic junction is especially susceptible to injury because it is a transition zone from the mobile to the rigid segment of the spinal cord.**
Cervical spine cord injuries are really very rare (< 50 per million per annum). The spinal canal in the cervical region is very spacious, so relatively large displacements of the vertebra of the cervical spine can occur without compromise to the spinal cord itself. The cervical spine is very mobile in several planes and so there is very little bony stability. Instead, the stability is provided by the ligaments connecting the motion segments. In contrast, the thoracic spine is relatively rigid. The transition between mobile and stiff segments in any mechanical structure is the area most vulnerable to extreme loads, and so the cervicothoracic junction (the area most difficult to visualize) is also the very area most likely to be fractured or dislocated.

45. **(c). Kidney—due to release of muscle degradation products**
As the patient rewarms and the limbs start to reperfuse, there is a real risk of myoglobin (released from damaged muscle) which will block the kidneys unless a rapid diuresis is started as soon as possible. No other organ is primarily at risk in the same way after crush syndrome.

46. **(c). Entry via neuronal and mucosal alpha (α) receptors**
The SARS-CoV2 invades the nervous tissue through ACE-2 or TMPRSS-2 and NOT through alpha (α) receptors.

47. **(b). Cervical cord compression**
Cervical cord compression leading to quadriplegia is a rare complication of the sitting position. Focal pressure on the spinal cord due to extreme flexion of the head on the neck is a postulated mechanism. Regional cord perfusion may also be decreased especially when there is associated decrease in MAP and could contribute to cord ischemia. Preventive measures could include avoidance of extreme flexion of the neck and providing a space of at least one inch between the chin and the chest, avoidance of excessive neck rotation particularly in elderly patients with cervical stenosis and maintenance of near normal MAP. Monitoring of short latency SSEPs have been advocated to monitor the sensory pathways during the procedure.

48. **(d). Inadequate analgesia may present similarly to delirium.**
    - Adequate postoperative analgesia reduces delirium
    - Pain should remain as a differential diagnosis in an elderly patient presenting with delirium

49. **(c). Behavioral changes**
This is True. Changes in human behavior like dressing warmly or adjusting ambient temperature are the most effective responses to changes in body temperature. The emotional distress of being too hot or too cold is commonly a significant factor in motivating human behavior to seek or produce an ambient temperature that is more "comfortable".

50. **(a). Preterm infants less than 37 weeks gestational age are excluded from the guidelines**
In the United States, the Guidelines for the determination of brain death in children exclude preterm infants less than 37 weeks because some of the brainstem reflexes are not completely developed in this group. Furthermore, the assessment of loss of consciousness in critically ill sedated and intubated neonates is difficult.

51. **(d). Patients with intraoperative hyperglycemia during neurosurgical procedures are more likely to develop postoperative neurologic dysfunction.**
In a retrospective examination of 1000 patients from the intraoperative hypothermia for aneurysm surgery trial database (IHAST) who underwent aneurysm clipping within 14 days of SAH, Pasternak et al. noted that at 3 months after surgery, those with glucose >129 mg/dL were more likely to have impaired cognition and those with glucose >152 mg/dL were more likely to experience gross neurologic dysfunction as assessed by the national institute of health stroke scale.

52. **(b). Phenylephrine is preferred for treating hypotension**
    Phenylephrine is preferred for treating hypotension. Through its alpha-agonist properties, phenylephrine increases SVR and maintains CPP without increasing chronotropy or inducing tachycardia. Phenylephrine has been used to treat intraoperative hypotension in patients with severe AS, it can restore the blood pressure to baseline rapidly without a significant decrease in cardiac output or impairment in systolic or diastolic function.

53. **(d). Control blood pressure to reduce intraoperative nose bleeding**
    Transsphenoidal pituitary surgery (TPS) can be intensely stimulating and thus leads to intraoperative hypertension. Significant hypertension may worsen intraoperative nose bleeding, which subsequently interferes with surgical exposure and visualization under microscope or endoscope during TPS.

54. **(d). When administered in doses sufficient to produce an isoelectric EEG, barbiturates decrease the cerebral metabolic rate for oxygen by 50%**
    When the EEG became isoelectric, a point at which cerebral metabolic activity is roughly 50% of baseline, no further decreases in $CMRO_2$ occurred. These findings support the hypothesis that metabolism and function of the brain are coupled. The effect of barbiturates on cerebral metabolism is maximized at a 50% depression of cerebral function, thus leaving all metabolic energy for the maintenance of cellular integrity.

55. **(c). Pain**

56. **(d). At least 48 hours prior**
    The efficacy of steroids in reducing cerebral edema associated with brain tumors (and only tumors) is well confirmed. Although the onset of this effect is relatively rapid, it is too slow for the management of acute intraoperative events. However, administration beginning 48 hours before an elective surgical procedure has the potential to reduce edema formation and improve the clinical condition by the time of craniotomy.

57. **(c). In a situation of low blood pressure, mannitol is preferable**
    Mannitol can lead to diuresis and volume depletion aggravating hypovolemia. Hypertonic saline may be the osmotic therapy of choice in hypovolemic or hypotensive patients because it remains in the intravascular space, thereby expanding intravascular volume and increasing MAP.

58. **(a). Hemolytic transfusion reaction**
    Hemolytic transfusion reactions are not the likely cause of lung infiltrates as in the above case. They usually manifest as bleeding diathesis, hypotension and hemoglobinuria. The classic signs and symptoms of a hemolytic transfusion reaction which are chills, fever, chest and flank pain, and nausea are masked by anesthesia. Intravascular hemolysis occurs when there is a direct attack on transfused donor cells by recipient antibody and complement. Treatment consists of prevention of kidney failure and a coagulopathy (DIC).

59. **(a). Vasodilation**
    Patients with spinal cord injury above the T4 level are at high-risk of the development of neurogenic shock. The patient suffers a sympathectomy, resulting in unopposed vagal tone. This leads to a distributive shock with hypotension and bradycardia. The loss of sympathetic tone results in vasodilation and inability to redirect blood flow from the periphery to the core circulation. Bradycardia is a characteristic finding of neurogenic shock and may help to differentiate from other forms of shock. Treatment requires fluid resuscitation as the first step (often referred to as "filling the tank") followed by pressors and inotropes.

60. **(c). They blunt the cerebrovascular response to CO_2**
    Cerebrovascular reactivity to CO_2 (vasodilation with hypercapnia and vasoconstriction with hypocapnia) has been considered to be regulated by the change in extracellular H^+ concentration mediated by nitric oxide, prostanoids, cyclic nucleotides, and intracellular calcium and potassium channel activity. At clinical levels of anesthesia, cerebrovascular responses to alterations in $PaCO_2$ are preserved with the use of inhalational agents, although the magnitude of response may vary according to the agent and anesthetic depth.

61. **(c). Propofol**
    In neurologically normal patients, autoregulation is preserved with intravenous anesthetics like propofol. This finding may be due, in part, to the vasoconstrictive effect of IV anesthetics.

62. **(d). Change of $PaCO_2$ from 40 to 60 mm Hg**
    Within the physiologic range of 20–60 mm Hg, CBF changes by 3–4% per 1 mm Hg change in CO_2 tension, with an accompanied commensurate change in CBV (cerebral blood volume). CO_2 reactivity is brisk and occurs within seconds of changing the arterial $PaCO_2$.

    A prolonged change in systemic CO_2 tension is accompanied by active transport of bicarbonate in or out of CSF to restore a normal acid-base balance (at 6 hours).

    Thus, the effects of hyperventilation on CBF are not sustained.

63. **(d). High dose steroids**
    National Acute Spinal Cord Injury Studies (NASCIS) trials. NASCIS II concluded there was efficacy of high-dose methylprednisolone in patients who had received the drug within 8 hours after injury. However, there are increased complications, such as pneumonia and gastrointestinal bleeding in patients treated with steroids. Based on these circumstances, the most recent version of the American Association of Neurological Surgeons and the Congress of Neurological Surgeons' Guidelines for the Management of Acute Cervical Spine and Spinal Cord Injuries state: "Administration of methylprednisolone (MP) for the treatment of acute SCI is not recommended".

64. **(c). Oral vitamin K_1**
    When there is a need for urgent anticoagulation reversal, warfarin should be discontinued and reversal of anticoagulation should occur immediately. Patients should first receive 2.5–10 mg of intravenous (IV) vitamin K_1 over a 30-minute period. This allows the liver, which may be depleted of vitamin K_1 and its associated coagulation factors, to synthesize vitamin K-dependent coagulation factors. However, this synthesis can take up to 24 hours. Oral vitamin K would take too long to work in this situation.

65. **(c). Micro-adenomas are usually nonfunctioning and detected incidentally**
    Micro-adenomas are <10 mm in diameter and present with hormonal excess (functional) and therefore are detected in the early stage. For example, Cushing's disease (excess ACTH).

66. **(c). Large pituitary adenoma**
    Although, most pituitary surgery is now done by transsphenoidal approach, transcranial approach may be indicated if the tumor is large or when there is little or no intrasellar tumor or the transsphenoidal approach has failed.

67. **(b). ECG changes**
    A significant VAE will manifest as RV strain pattern and ST depression on the ECG and they manifest along with hemodynamic instability which is a late sign.

68. **(c). Midazolam and fentanyl have minimal effects on EP recordings**
    Opioids and benzodiazepines have negligible effects on EP monitoring.

69. **(a). Vasospasm can be detected as early as 3 hours of SAH**
    Studies using TCD ultrasonography have confirmed the delayed onset and time course of vasospasm. Evidence of vasospasm initially was seen 3 days after SAH, appeared to be maximal between days 6 and 8, and was much reduced by day 12. It is unlikely for vasospasm to be evident within 3 hours.

70. **(a). Anti-Parkinson's medications should be given the morning of surgery**
    Patients undergoing deep brain stimulation have their medications stopped 12 hours before the procedure for assessment of physiological recordings and behavioral responses after placement of the stimulation electrode in the brain.

71. **(b). Rapid lowering of blood pressure to prevent bleeding**
    After an acute stroke rapid lowering of blood pressure could prove harmful. Nicardipine and/or labetalol should be used to keep MAP <140 mm Hg.

72. **(c). C4 cervical nerve root**
    The greater occipital nerve arises from C2 and innervates the posterior scalp.

73. **(d). Unilateral visual field defect**
    Upward enlargement of the pituitary gland leads to compression of the optic chiasma and leads to visual field defects and decreased visual acuity. Bitemporal hemianopia occurs in 75% of the patients.

74. **(a). Most of the transport of glucose in brain requires energy**
    GLUT1 receptors expressed in endothelial cells which are part of the blood brain barrier and GLUT3 in neurons are responsible for transporting glucose into the brain through the process of facilitated diffusion. These transporters move glucose down its concentration gradient (from higher to lower concentration), a process which does not require energy.

75. **(b). Fentanyl**
    Opioids are commonly used in anesthesia in part to suppress hypothalamic and pituitary hormone secretion. Morphine suppresses the release of corticotrophin from the hypothalamus and has also been found to inhibit cortisol release. In cardiac surgery Fentanyl, Sufentanil, and Alfentanil suppress pituitary hormone secretion ultimately limiting glucose production.

76. **(b). Hypocarbia is a precipitating factor**
    Hypercarbia rather than hypocarbia is a risk factor for the development of TCR. Other risk factors are light anesthesia, hypoxia, and acidosis.

77. **(b). It uses SHANON equation**

78. **(c). A-4, B-3, C-2, D-1**

Band	Frequency range
Alpha	7–13 Hz
Beta	13–30 Hz
Beta 2/Gamma	30–50 Hz
Theta	3.5–7 Hz
Delta	0.5–3.5 Hz

79. **(a). 17°C**
    Cerebral metabolic rate decreases by 6–7% per degree celsius of temperature reduction. In addition to anesthetic drugs, hypothermia can also cause complete suppression of the EEG (at approximately 18–20°C).

80. **(c). Preemptive atropine**
    This is false. Prophylactic administration of atropine or glycopyrrolate preoperatively does not provide protection against development of TCR.
    Cholinergic blockade reduces but does not totally prevent the lowering of the HR or BP.

81. **(c). It predominantly occurs in patients who have coronary artery disease**
    Coronary artery spasm can occur in patients undergoing neurosurgical procedures in the vicinity of the trigeminal nerve with no cardiac history. Most of the events are transient but can progress to myocardial infarction, ventricular fibrillation and asystole if the inciting factor is not removed or with improper management.

82. **(c). 3rd trimester**
    The risk of rupture for both AVMs and aneurysms is highest in the 3rd trimester. Incidence of hemorrhage increases with advanced gestation, possibly due to increases in cardiac output or, possibly, from hormonal influences on vascular integrity.

83. **(b). Parturients with tethered cord**
    Spinal anesthesia for adult tethered cord syndrome (TCS) should be avoided because it can cause complex neurological complications. When a patient has mild symptoms such as back pain, neurogenic bladder, motor, or sensory change, it is extremely important for the anesthesiologist to be aware of the possibility of TCS. When acute onset of paresthesia or weakness in the lower extremities occurs after surgery, MRI should be promptly performed to make the diagnosis.

84. **(a). It is a noninvasive measurement of regional cerebral oxygenation**
    While brain tissue oxygen tension monitoring is a focal and invasive monitor, cerebral oximetry is noninvasive global monitor of regional cerebral perfusion.

85. **(d). Current evidence for antipsychotic prophylaxis for POD is insufficient**
    There is limited, contradictory and inconsistent support in literature to support prophylactic use of antipsychotics like haloperidol, for prevention of POD. There is more potential harm than benefit, like CNS effects (such as somnolence, extrapyramidal effects such as muscle rigidity, tremor, restlessness, swallowing difficulty, decreased seizure threshold, and neuroleptic malignant syndrome), systemic and cardiovascular effects (such as QT prolongation, dysrhythmias, sudden death, hypotension, and tachycardia).

86. **(c). Acute fulminant hepatic failure is a common cause of encephalopathy**
    Acute fulminant failure is fatal but not a common cause of encephalopathy. Cerebral edema and brain herniation is usually the cause of death. Cytotoxic effects of ammonia, glutamine, cytokines and disruption of the blood brain barrier lead to increased ICP.

87. **(d). Dexmedetomidine**
    Recent evidence has demonstrated the anti-apoptotic effect of dexmedetomidine in different brain injury models. It was found to prevent cortical apoptosis in vitro and in vivo and attenuate isoflurane-induced injury in the developing brain, providing neurocognitive protection.

88. **(d). Multimodal monitoring would better help to guide individual therapy following TBI**
    Multimodal neuromonitoring helps in assessment of cerebral hemodynamics, oxygenation, and metabolic status and allows for individually tailored approach to management and prevention of secondary ischemic brain injury. After injury: in this patient treatment decisions can be guided by monitoring changes in physiologic variables rather than by predefined, generic thresholds.

89. **(d). The bioavailability of intranasal route is 90%.**
    The bioavailability of the intranasal (IN) route is 50%

90. **(a). It takes 2 hours for hyperventilation to become clinically effective**
    The CBF decrease and consequent vasoconstrictive effect of hyperventilation and hypocapnia occurs within minutes.

91. **(b). Reverse Trendelenburg position**
    If a venous air embolism is suspected, placing the patient in a head down (Trendelenburg) position helps prevent further air entry into the venous circulation, while also helping to prevent more air entering the pulmonary circulation by trapping air in the apex of the right ventricle.

92. **(c). Induced hypothermia**
    Induced hypothermia would not be recommended during acute rupture of an intracranial aneurysm. Hypothermia can cause harm like cardiac arrhythmias, platelets function defects and bacteremia. There are no high quality studies supporting the use of induced hypothermia in this situation.

93. **(a). Ischemic optic neuropathy (ION) is associated with emboli into the retinal artery**
    Prone and Trendelenburg position increase intraocular pressure and ophthalmic vein congestion leading to ION.

Central retinal artery occlusion is caused by emboli of the retinal artery.

94. **(d). Hyperventilation for raised ICP should only be used for a brief period**
Hyperventilation is routinely used to provide brain relaxation and optimize surgical conditions.
However, the decrease CBF from hyperventilation-induced cerebral vasoconstriction can potentially cause or exacerbate cerebral ischemia.

95. **(b). Pyramidal cells**
EEG recorded with the help of scalp electrode, is the summation of multiple post synaptic potentials (inhibitory and excitatory) generated by pyramidal cell in the cortex of the brain.

96. **(d). Awakening of anesthesia**
On emergence from anesthesia, the alpha oscillations transition to lower amplitude beta and gamma oscillations. At the same time, the slow and delta oscillations dissipate. The loss of the alpha and slow-delta oscillation power again appears in the spectrogram as a zipper opening pattern.

97. **(a). Time domain analysis**
Ways of analysis of EEG waveform consist of: Time domain analysis, freqeuncy domain analysis, phase domain analysis. Burst suppression is characteristic feature seen in time domain analysis.

98. **(d). Noninvasive focal oxygenation**
Near infrared spectroscopy (NIRS) is a noninvasive assessment of oxygenation within the human brain (SCO_2) by appreciating the different absorption of near infrared light by hemoglobin and oxyhemoglobin. It is based on modified Beer-Lambert law. The depth of assessment is dependent on the distance between to light source and sensors.

99. **(a). 25 : 75**
Most NIRS devices use a fixed reference ratio between the arterial (25%) and venous contribution (75%). This assumption is based on anatomical evidence.

100. **(c). Blood flow velocity in brain circulation**
Transcranial Doppler ultrasonography calculates the velocity of red blood cells (FV) by means of the Doppler principle. The change in the frequency of emitted pulse of ultrasound reflected by red blood cells is proportional to blood flow velocity. By convention, the shift in Doppler frequency is expressed in centimeters per second.

101. **(a). 2 MHz**
Transcranial Doppler ultrasonography calculates the velocity of red blood cells (FV) by means of the Doppler principle. The frequency best suited for TCD applications is on the order of 2 MHz.

102. **(c). Intraventricular catheter**
- The intraventricular technique is accurate but requires cannulation of one of the ventricular frontal horns. CSF infection, overshunting, and intraparenchymal and intraventricular hemorrhages are among the most common complications associated with this technique.
- Intraparenchymal techniques rely on technical variations of the strain gauge method. Zeroing is performed once, prior to intraparenchymal insertion of the sensor, and the catheter is held in place by a variety of devices, the most popular being the bolt screw. This method is user friendly, requires minimal maintenance, and is easily movable during patient transport.

103. **(d). Marshall's grade**
- World Federation of Neurosurgical Society (WFNS): they 5 grades on the basis of GCS and motor deficits
- *Modified Fischer grade:* This system is used to grade SAH. Higher the grade poorer the outcome
- *Hunt and Hess grade:* It was developed to predict prognosis and outcome in patients with SAH. It is based on patients presenting symptoms
- *Marshalls grade*: It was developed to grade severity of diffuse axonal edema.

104. **(b). Andexanet alpha**
Andexanet alfa is a recombinant factor Xa protein used for reversal of apixaban and rivaroxaban in patients with life-threatening or uncontrolled bleeding approved by the FDA in May 2018.

105. **(c). Vertebral column**
Denis divided the vertebral column into 3 vertical parallel columns.
Instability occurs when injuries affect 2 contiguous columns.
Anterior column consisted of anterior longitudinal ligament, anterior two-thirds of the vertebral body, anterior two-thirds of the intervertebral disk. Middle column consist of posterior one-third of the vertebral body and the associated intervertebral disk, posterior longitudinal ligament (PLL). Posterior column consists of everything posterior to the PLL.

106. **(a). Tranexamic acid**
CRASH-3 evaluated the role of tranexamic acid for patients with traumatic brain injury. Approximately 10000 patients were recruits. Study group received 1 g bolus of tranexamic acid (TNX) followed 1 infusion over 8 hours within 3 hours of injury. Subgroup analysis showed that people with mild-to-moderate injury (GCS 9-15) had maximum benefit from TNX. It is technically a negative trial as the primary endpoints did not reach statistically significant results.

107. **(d). Entropy < 50**
Triple low concept was first defined by Sessler et al. It refers to a intraoperative state where there is hypotension, low MAC and low BIS value. Sessler et al. showed that triple low is associated with higher 30 day perioperative mortality risk.

108. **(c). Vasogenic edema**
Vasogenic edema is associated with disruption of blood brain barrier secondary to mechanical damage due like brain trauma or chemical mediators following tumors, infection.
Cytotoxic edema is seen in cases with disrupted ionic pump with anaerobic metabolism' which is either due to ischemia or hypoxia.
Interstitial edema, also known as hydrocephalic edema, is cause due to breakdown of ventricular ependymal lining in hydrocephalus leading to transependymal migration of CSF into the surrounding space.
Osmotic edema is seen in patients with imbalance between serum and brain osmolarity.

109. **(a). 3rd nerve compression**
A dilated, unresponsive pupil may be a sign of ipsilateral herniation of medial aspect of the temporal lobe (uncus) through the tentorium, thereby compressing the midbrain and nucleus of the third cranial nerve.

110. **(d). Cherry red macula is seen in ION**
Postoperative visual loss is a rare but dreaded complication seen mostly in patients getting operated in prone position. Many differentials have been described, most common being ION, central retinal artery occlusion (CRAO). CRAO is associated with classical diagnostic finding of cherry red macula with white ground glass appearance of retina.

111. **(d). 140 mEq/L.**
Each 1,000 mL of PL 148 contains 5.26 g sodium chloride, 370 mg potassium chloride, 300 mg magnesium chloride, 3.68 g and 5.02 g of sodium acetate and sodium gluconate respectively; this equates to 140 mmol/L sodium, 5 mmol/L potassium, 1.5 mmol/L magnesium, 98 mmol/L chloride, and 27 mmol/L and 23 mmol/L of acetate and gluconate, respectively.

112. **(b). Factor X a**
Rivaroxaban, apixaban and edoxaban are direct inhibitors of factor X a. dabigatran is a direct inhibitor of Factor II a (Direct Thrombin Inhibitors)

113. **(d). CRASH**
- ENIGMA: Evaluated the role nitrous oxide in major surgeries
- IMPACT: Randomized, multicenter study comparing the efficacy and safety of fluticasone furoate/umeclidinium/vilanterol (FF/UMEC/VI) vs FF/VI and UMEC/VI in patients ≥40 years of age with symptomatic COPD and a history of exacerbations
- CRASH: Placebo-controlled trial to assess the effects of a 48-hour infusion of corticosteroids on death and on neurological disability, among adults with head injury
- DECRA: Multi-center randomized trial to evaluate the effect of early decompressive craniectomy on neurological function in patients with severe traumatic brain injury.

114. **(a). Anterior atlantodental interval (ADI) greater than 5 mm**
Atlantoaxial dislocation (AAD) can be defined with radiographic measurements of atlantoaxial joint articulation using the ADI. The ADI is a small slit like space between the posterior aspect of the anterior atlas ring and the anterior aspect of the odontoid process. Flexion and extension radiographs of the neck is used for measurement of the ADI and to determine whether the atlantoaxial joint reduces itself in these positions. The ADI is normally constant in distance during movement of the head and generally does not exceed 5 mm for adults and 3 mm for children

115. **(b). More common in males**
Myasthenia gravis (MG) is an autoimmune disorder in which antibodies bind to acetylcholine receptors or related molecules. Ice-pack test is used to diagnose MG as its application reverses ptosis. It is treated with thymectomy, immunosuppression and in certain severe cases with plasmapheresis. Autoimmune disease are more common in female.

116. **(c). Surfactant is secreted by type IV pneumocytes.**

117. **(a). *Escherichia coli, Enterobacteria***
- *Escherichia coli, Enterobacteria* are lactose fermenting species which will grow pink colonies
- *Salmonella, Proteus, Yersinia* will form white colonies due to absence of lactose fermentation.
- *Staphylococci* will not form any colonies on MacConkey medium
- *Acid fast bacilli do not grow on* MacConkey medium.

118. **(c). Lung compliance in decreased**
In emphysema, the slope of the pressure-volume curve is steeper indicting increased compliance. However it does not decrease work of breathing due to increased airway resistance.

119. **(c). They are resistant to fourth generation cephalosporin's like cefepime**
ESBL are gram negative. Sensitive to cephamycins and resistant to cephalosporins including fourth generation cefepime. They are intrinsically sensitive to carbapenems.

120. **(d). Continuous Positive Airway Pressure (CPAP) Therapy increases FRC.**

121. **(d). Check pulse and blood pressure**
    Monitor shows ventricular tachycardia (VT). The treatment of pulseless VT is defibrillation. VT with pulse if hemodynamically unstable, needs synchronized cardioversion. VT with pulse, if hemodynamically stable, is treated with chemical cardioversion (Amiodarone 150 mg IV over 15 minutes).

122. **(c). Change of compressor every 5 minutes of compressions**
    Change of compressor every 2 minutes of compressions is recommended for high quality CPR.

123. **(c). Underdamped system**
    Rapidly flushing the arterial line by pilling the flush device generates a square form.
    Normally, 2 oscillations are seen in optimally functioning arterial waveform. Less than 1.5 oscillations indicate overdamping, and will read false low systolic BP. Oscillations more than 2 indicate underdamping, which shows false high systolic BP. In either cases the mean arterial pressure remains unaffected.

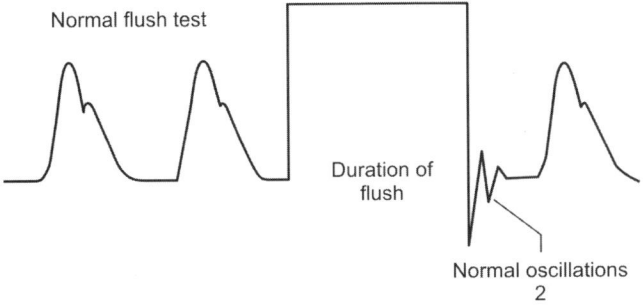

124. **(a). Nitrous oxide is not flammable at atmospheric pressure**
    Nitrous oxide is not flammable. An anesthetic machine should be connected to a conducting floor of an operating theatre to prevent the production of static electrical sparks. A current of approximately 100 microamperes is needed to produce a microshock to the heart, capable of producing ventricular fibrillation. Since all connections have some finite resistance the neutral connection is not exactly at earth potential at the patient end of the circuit. The heat released in surgical diathermy depends on the resistance and to the square of the current flowing.

125. **(c). 20% of the combined sensory-motor neuropathy result in permanent motor dysfunction and pain**
    80% of the combined sensory-motor neuropathy result in permanent motor dysfunction and pain.

126. **(d). Normal waveform seen in advanced pregnancy**
    Pigtail capnogram is seen in advanced pregnancy, obese individuals and poor lung compliance. It is due to the sudden peak of pre-inspiratory expired CO_2 secondary to sudden airway closure. It occurs when a poorly compliant lung, central obesity or a term pregnant abdomen leads to escape of few milliliters of CO_2-rich gas from the alveoli before small airway closure.

127. **(b). Factors XI, XIII, antithrombin III, protein S, platelets decrease while II, V, protein C levels remain unchanged**
    Pregnancy is hypercoagulable state with gestational thrombocytopenia. Maximum increase is with factors I & VII, lesser increase in VIII, IX, X, XII von Willebrand factor, 20% decrease in PT, PTT, and decrease in factors XI, XIII, antithrombin III, protein S with no change in II, V and protein C levels.

128. **(c). Dural puncture with 25 gauge spinal needle using "needle-through-needle" technique after locating epidural with epidural needle with no medication into the intrathecal space**
    Dural puncture epidural. After the epidural space is located with the epidural needle, a pencil-point spinal needle is inserted utilizing the "needle-through-needle" technique and the dura is punctured. A 25- or 26-gauge spinal needle is usually used because a DPE placed by a 27-gauge needle was shown to offer no benefit in a single study. No medication is directly introduced into the intrathecal space but the dural puncture may facilitate the intrathecal migration of medication administered into the epidural space.

129. **(b). Hypertension**
    Potential causes of maternal cardiac arrest are:
    A: Anesthetic complications, B: Bleeding C: Cardiac, D: Drugs, E: Embolism, F: Fetal, G: General nonobstetric causes of cardiac arrest, H: Hypertension.

130. **(d). 12–24 weeks postpartum**
    Cardiac output decreases to just below prelabor values at 24 hours postpartum, and returns to prepregnancy levels 12–24 weeks postpartum.

131. **(c). Increased PaO_2, decreased $PaCO_2$ and HCO_3 with pH towards alkalotic side**
    During pregnancy, PaO_2 increases to 100–105 mm Hg as a result of greater alveolar ventilation and there is a decline in $PaCO_2$ to approximately 30 mm Hg. The respiratory alkalosis of pregnancy causes a compensatory increase in renal bicarbonate excretion causing serum HCO_3 to decrease to 20 mEq/L and an elevation of pH by 0.02–0.06 units.

132. **(a). Increased sleep time, decreased stage 3 and 4 NREM in 1st trimester with decreased REM and total sleep in 3rd trimester**

Sleep characteristics change as pregnancy progresses. The American Academy of Sleep medicine defined pregnancy associated sleep disorder as the occurrence of insomnia or excessive sleepiness that develops in the course of pregnancy.

133. **(c). Initial force of 10 N when patient is awake increased to 30 N as patient becomes unconscious**

134. **(c). Propofol, thiopentone, ketamine**
Atropine, propofol, thiopentone, ketamine, ephedrine, nitroglycerin cross the placental barrier.

135. **(d). Epinephrine**
Atropine is not preferred. Glycopyrrolate is contraindicated in neonates due to benzyl alcohol.

136. **(c). 1.5 mL/kg bolus followed by 0.25 mL/kg/min infusion not exceeding 12 mL/kg**

137. **(d). Epinephrine in lower doses than normal and avoiding vasopressin**

138. **(d). Subdural space**
Subdural injection of local anesthetic is associated with high patchy blockade, intermediate onset time, cranial nerve involvement with no sacral analgesia, apnea, unconsciousness, Horner's syndrome, less motor blockade and hypotension than with high or total spinal anesthesia.

139. **(a). Four hours or more in nulliparous women, 3 hours or more in parous women**
Definition of second-stage arrest is no progress (descent or rotation) for:
- Four hours or more in nulliparous women with epidural analgesia
- Three hours or more in nulliparous women without epidural analgesia
- Three hours or more in parous women with epidural analgesia
- Two hours or more in parous women without epidural analgesia.

140. **(c). Rapid sequence spinal for Category 1 caesarean section**
'Rapid Sequence Spinal' involves:
- Deploy other staff to secure the intravenous line
- Preoxygenate during the attempt
- 'No Touch Technique' use only gloves, chlorhexidine on swab to paint and use glove packet as sterile surface
- Local injection not mandatory
- Add 25 mcg fentanyl, if there is time. If not consider increasing the dose of bupivacaine
- Only one attempt at spinal unless obvious correction allows a successful second attempt
- Start surgery once sensory level >T10 and ascending. Be ready for general anesthesia and inform the mother.

141. **(a). Phenylephrine or ephedrine**
A randomized trial of phenylephrine and ephedrine in treating hypotension in preeclamptics with LSCS under SA showed no differences between groups in umbilical artery and vein base excess values or Apgar scores. The NICE guidelines state that both are equally effective as vasopressors.

142. **(b). Phenylephrine has decreased uterine vascular resistance as compared to ephedrine**

143. **(a). During PCA, a high ratio of patient demands to delivered bolus doses, signifies adequate pain relief**
During PCA, the ratio of patient demands to delivered bolus doses appears to be a good measure of analgesia and is strongly correlated with pain scores. A high ratio reflects patient misunderstanding or inadequate analgesia and a ratio closer to 1 signifies adequate pain relief.

144. **(a). Once the balloon catheter is placed, flexion of the hips during positioning for a neuraxial anesthetic technique is discouraged, because it may result in balloon dislodgement or occlusion and subsequent thrombosis**
The placement of an epidural catheter before an intravascular balloon catheter is preferred for the following reasons:
- Once the balloon catheter is placed, flexion of the hips (during positioning for a neuraxial anesthetic technique) is discouraged, because it may result in balloon dislodgement or occlusion and subsequent thrombosis;
- Epidural anesthesia seems preferable to the use of local anesthesia with sedation for balloon catheter placement;
- During balloon catheter placement, small amounts of heparin are sometimes used, and it seems preferable to have the epidural catheter in place before anticoagulation; and
- Should untoward events (e.g., fetal compromise, vessel rupture) occur during the procedure, the epidural catheter allows for rapid extension of anesthesia for cesarean delivery.

145. **(a). Meperidine is recommended in obstetric patients due to longer duration of action and no effect on fetus**
Meperidine is avoided in obstetric patients because of the accumulation of normeperidine in the neonate and its subsequent effect on neurobehavioral scores.

146. **(a). Gestational hypertension: 20 weeks gestational age to 12 weeks postpartum, proteinuria present**
There is no proteinuria in gestational hypertension.

147. **(a). Maternal insulin requirements decrease with the onset of labor, increase again during the second stage of labor**
    - Maternal insulin requirements decrease with the onset of labor, increase again during the second stage of labor, and decrease markedly during the early postpartum period
    - Intravenous glucose and insulin infusions during the peripartum period should be titrated to maintain a maternal blood glucose concentration of 70–90 mg/L (3.9 – 5 mmol/L)
    - Diabetic scleredema can lead to anterior spinal artery syndrome after neuraxial anesthesia by reducing epidural space due to noncompliant connective tissue. Hence lower volumes are suggested
    - Pregnancy may accelerate the development of proliferative retinopathy, a microvascular complication of DM, pregnancy does not accelerate the progression of diabetic nephropathy

148. **(d). As per recent studies respiratory depression after neuraxial morphine administration is triphasic- immediate dose dependent, delayed due to rostral spread, late onset during dissociation phase**
    - Respiratory monitoring after neuraxial administration of morphine should occur at least every hour for the first 12 hours and then every 2 hours for the next 12 hours
    - Respiratory monitoring after administration of neuraxial fentanyl should continue for a minimum of 2 hours
    - Early-onset respiratory depression associated with lipophilic opioids usually occurs within 30 minutes of administration
    - Respiratory depression after neuraxial morphine administration is biphasic – early due to vascular absorption and delayed due to rostral spread.

149. **(a). Opioid-induced histamine release from mast cells appears to be one of the causative mechanism for pruritus after neuraxial opioid administration**
    - Opioid-induced histamine release from mast cells does not appear to be the causative mechanism for pruritus after neuraxial opioid administration
    - Pregnant patients may be more susceptible as a result of estrogen interaction with opioid receptors
    - There may be a genetic predisposition to pruritus due to opioid receptor genotype
    - Pentazocine, a κ-opioid receptor agonist and partial μ-opioid receptor agonist, may be a useful drug for treating opioid-induced pruritus.

150. **(c). Oxytocin: Malignant hyperthermia**
Oxytocin: Malignant hyperthermia. It can be safely administered.

151. **(d). Sugammadex, unlike neuromuscular blocking agents, has high placental transfer rates**
    - Dantrolene crosses the placenta and may result in neonatal hypotonia if administered before delivery.
    - Dabigatran, a reversible thrombin inhibitor, crosses the placenta with an F/M ratio of 0.33.
    - Sodium nitroprusside is lipid soluble, rapidly crosses the placenta, and can produce cyanide as a byproduct
    - Sugammadex, which directly binds and reverses the neuromuscular blockade of steroidal muscle relaxants, has low placental transfer rates.

152. **(c). A-WHITACRE, B-QUINCKE, C-PITKIN, D-SPROTTE**

153. **(c). Indomethacin causes maternal platelet dysfunction and so is a contraindication for neuraxial anesthesia**
    - Atosiban is an oxytocin receptor antagonist. It is a competitive inhibitor of oxytocin that binds to both myometrial and decidual receptors. Associated with higher rate of perinatal deaths
    - Nifedipine can cause vasodilation, hypotension, myocardial depression, and conduction defects when used in combination with volatile halogenated anesthetic agents
    - Indomethacin causes transient fetal ductal constriction, tricuspid regurgitation, oligohydramnios and maternal platelet dysfunction but no contraindication for neuraxial anesthesia
    - Terbutaline has resulted in the following maternal side effects:
        - Hypotension;
        - Tachycardia, with or without cardiac arrhythmias and myocardial ischemia;
        - Pulmonary edema;
        - Hyperglycemia; and
        - Hypokalemia.

154. **(c). As the name suggests, it is always reversible with treatment**
Irreversible cytotoxic edema with permanent neurologic damage can occur if the initial disorder is not diagnosed early.

155. **(d). Paradoxical oxytocin headache**

156. **(a). Onset of heart failure during the last month of pregnancy or within 5 months of delivery with no other identifiable cause of heart failure and no known heart disease before pregnancy**

- Onset of heart failure during the last month of pregnancy or within 5 months of delivery with no other identifiable cause of heart failure and no known heart disease before pregnancy
- Onset of heart failure before the last month of pregnancy with no other identifiable cause of heart failure and no known heart disease before pregnancy is called pregnancy-associated cardiomyopathy
- Pregnancy-associated dynamic left ventricular outflow tract obstruction with obstruction gradient typically increasing after a premature ventricular contraction associated with pregnancy is hypertrophic cardiomyopathy
- Potentially reversible condition associated with rapid atrial or ventricular rates caused by arrhythmias in pregnancy is tachycardia induced cardiomyopathy.

157. (d). 1-C, 2-A, 3-D, 4-B

158. (a). **Oxytocin does not require cold chain, hence recommended in low resource setups**
Oxytocin needs cold chain maintenance.

159. (c). **Nicardipine is now recommended as a first-line agent in women for whom intravenous access is difficult to secure**
In the absence of contraindications, nifedipine is now recommended as a first-line agent in women for whom intravenous access is difficult to secure.

160. (c). **Measures to lower fetal mortality include hypothermic cardiopulmonary bypass with flow rates >2.4 L/min/m² while maintaining mean arterial blood pressure above 70–75 mm Hg.**
Measures to lower fetal mortality include **normothermic** cardiopulmonary bypass with flow rates greater than 2.4 L/min/m² while maintaining mean arterial blood pressure above 70–75 mm Hg.

161. (b). **Magnesium sulfate is preferred to diazepam for the prevention of further seizures in eclampsia**
Neuraxial analgesia/anesthesia can be considered in stable eclamptic women (fully conscious, no recent seizures, treated with magnesium sulfate, and no organ failure).
Fetal bradycardia typically begins during or immediately after a seizure but does not mandate immediate delivery unless it is persistent.
Late eclampsia is defined as seizure onset from 48 hours after delivery to 4 weeks postpartum.

162. (d.) **ED90 is almost ten times lower, approximately 3 IU, in women undergoing cesarean delivery for labour arrest after labor augmentation or induction with oxytocin**
ED90 is almost ten times **higher**, approximately 3 IU, in women undergoing cesarean delivery for labor arrest after labor augmentation or induction with oxytocin.

163. (d). Femoral nerve

164. (d). **If the blood type is unknown and blood products are required immediately, type O Rh positive RBCs and type AB plasma can be administered to obstetric patients**
If the blood type is unknown and blood products are required immediately, type O Rh **negative** RBCs and type AB plasma can be administered.

165. (d). **Not to exceed 1 g administered slowly over 10 minutes; repeated once if bleeding continues after 30 minutes, followed by continuous infusion**
Continuous infusion is not recommended.
Administration beyond 3 hours does not confer clinical benefit (WHO recommendation).
Tranexamic acid crosses the placenta. Not to exceed 1 g administered slowly over 10 minutes; repeated once if bleeding continues after 30 minutes, followed by continuous infusion.

166. (d). **Normal value is always above 75%**
Normal values range from 60 to 80%; however, lower values of 55–60% are not considered abnormal in some cardiac patients. It is more important to follow trends rather than an absolute value.

167. (b). Respiratory rate
Parameters included in Apgar score are activity (tone), pulse (rate), grimace, colour, respiration. Respiratory rate (in breaths per minute) is not a feature.

168. (d). **Multiply exposed children did not show a decrease in motor skills, behavioral speed, processing and reading**

169. (b). C4

170. (c). Percutaneous tracheostomy

171. (b). **Uterine incision to cord-clamping interval should not exceed 3 minutes**
There is no time limit. The neonates' airway has to be secured, and following that the cord is clamped. Until then the oxygenation is maintained through placental circulation.

172. (b). **Fetal circulation is two circuits in parallel while adult circulation is in series**

173. (b). **Fasting guidelines should be followed if the child is stable**

174. (d). **Weight 10 lbs, age 10 weeks, Hb 10 gm/dL**

175. (c). Young children with OSA are generally obese

176. (a). 2-4 J/kg

177. (d). Loading dose of dantrolene for treatment is 1 mg/kg
    The dose of dantrolene is 2-2.5 mg/kg up to a maximum of 300 mg.

178. (b). The threshold PAED score to diagnose ED is ≥10
    The incidence is maximum in 1-5 years of age. Incidence with sevoflurane and desflurane is similar. Incidence with inhalational anesthesia is high 10-80%.

179. (b). 20 minutes

180. (b). Reduced tissue/gas solubility in the vessel rich group of tissues

181. (d). Neurological features precede cardiovascular collapse

182. (d). Coughing during open eye surgery can cause prolapse of intraocular contents

183. (c). Wake-up test during scoliosis surgery is contraindicated in children

184. (b). Facial burns are a warning of possible airway burns and inhalational injury

185. (c). It is not effective orally

186. (d). Is nearly always caused by a "lead point" such as a polyp or duplication

187. (d). Generally does not present until 1-2 months of life
    This condition presents at birth.

188. (d). The diagnosis is best made with a barium swallow.
    Barium swallow used to be done earlier. Nowadays diagnosis is best done using ultrasound.

189. (b). Contractility of the heart

190. (d). It is important to initiate beta blocker therapy before alpha blocker therapy to prevent side effects

191. (b). Avoid decrease in systemic vascular resistance and fast heart rate

192. (d). Greater ratio of alveolar ventilation to functional residual capacity

193. (b). Caudal administration of 0.125% bupivacaine is as effective as caudal administration of 0.25% bupivacaine

194. (b). Larger tongue relative to the oropharynx than in an adult

195. (c). Accurately assesses proprioceptive integrity

196. (a). The dural sac extends further caudad than in adults

197. (d). Monitor for apnea for 24 hours postoperatively
    Premature infants are prone to postoperative apnea till about 55-60 weeks post-conceptional age.

198. (d). None of the above

199. (c). 8

200. (c). 6-12 months of age
    MAC is low/minimum in premature neonates, high in term neonates till 6 months of age, and approximates adult values from 6 months onwards.

201. (b). Associated systemic congenital anomalies are very common

202. (b). Adenotonsillar hypertrophy

203. (a). Muscle relaxants

204. (c). Radiation

205. (a). DiGeorge syndrome

206. (b). Ropivacaine

207. (b). 55-70 mm Hg

208. (b). 90-100 mL/kg

209. (c). Diaphragm has predominantly type 1 muscle fibers

210. (b). High level disinfection

211. (c). PRISM score

212. (b). To assess gestational age in infants

213. (a). It helps determine the duration of action of a drug infusion after stopping the infusion

214. (d). Distance from the Y-piece to the terminal bronchioles

215. (b). When advancing the needle during TAP blocks, the needle tip is best seen with an in plane needle view

216. (d). It is the least potent among the currently used agents
    Desflurane is an inhalational agent with low solubility in blood and body tissues. It has a MAC of 6% and the lowest potency among the currently used volatile agents. It has a boiling point of 22.8°C. All volatile agents in current use are triggers for malignant hyperthermia and potentiate the action of muscle relaxants.

217. (d). Can cause hepatitis due to compound A formation
    Sevoflurane is a halogenated methyl-isopropyl ether and has a minimal alveolar concentration (MAC)

quoted at between approximately 2–2.5%. The boiling point of sevoflurane is 58.8°C and the saturated vapor pressure (SVP) is 157 mm Hg. Sevoflurane is 2% metabolized by the liver but forms no reactive products.

Compound A is formed by the reaction of sevoflurane with dry carbon dioxide absorbers at low gas flows, and is nephrotoxic not hepatotoxic. The formation of compound A is greater with carbon dioxide absorbers which contain sodium and potassium hydroxides. The fluoride ion is also produced by the metabolism of sevoflurane that is nephrotoxic in rats, although the significance to humans is debatable.

218. (d). TEC 7
Mechanical variable bypass vaporizers are prone to contamination of the bypass chamber with liquid agent if tilted. 1 mL of liquid provides 200 mL of vapor, which results in a significant overdose in the next breath. Aladin cassettes are detachable vaporizing units. The bypass chamber is within the working station, hence cannot be contaminated if the cassette is tilted. In injector vaporizers, there are no wicks to saturate and the liquid anesthetic reservoir and vaporizing chamber are separate. Hence, the liquid agent cannot spill into the vaporizing chamber.

219. (b). Conductors of electricity
Mechanical variable bypass vaporizers do not require electric power to function.

Metals have high specific heat and thermal conductivity. Metals like steel, brass, aluminium and copper are used in the construction of vaporizers to compensate for the loss of latent heat of vaporization. They are used as heat sinks and to conduct environmental heat to the liquid agent and also as thermostats (bimetallic strips, invar rod).

220. (d). $EtCO_2$
Capnography is conventionally expressed in mmHg. Other agents and gases including, oxygen, nitrogen and nitrous oxide are conventionally mentioned in v/v%.

221. (d). Desflurane
Desflurane is very volatile. It has a low boiling point (22.4°C) and high SVP (664 mm Hg) leading to rapid uncontrollable vaporization in the initial phase. When the liquid cools and vaporization falls the patient is at risk of awareness. This is compounded by low blood gas solubility (0.45) and high MAC (6%). Current workstations are unable to deliver adequate fresh gas flows to dilute the initial high output to clinically usable amounts. The temperature compensation mechanisms used in mechanical variable bypass vaporizers are accurate between 15–35°C. The output will be inaccurate when the temperature falls below this level.

222. (c). Oxford Miniature Vaporizer
The Oxford Miniature Vaporizer was designed in 1962. Changes in internal temperature as a result of the heat lost during vaporization are buffered by the presence of a water/ethylene glycol jacket.

The TEC and Dräger 2000 are mechanically temperature compensated with thermostats. The Aladin cassette vaporizer is electrically heated and electronically compensated.

223. (a). Halothane
Halothane is a halogenated hydrocarbon. $CF_3CHClBr$.

224. (d). Xenon
With a blood/gas partition coefficient of 0.115, xenon is the least soluble gas that may be used for anesthesia.

The blood/gas partition coefficients of the agents mentioned are as follows—desflurane (0.46), nitrous oxide (0.42) and Sevoflurane (0.65).

225. (c). Sevoflurane
Sevoflurane is susceptible to various types of chemical degradation. Most pertinent is the degradation of sevoflurane by Lewis acids (such as metal oxides and metal halides), to hydrofluoric acid, and to other toxic compounds. Hydrofluoric acid (HF), even in minute amounts, is highly reactive, corrosive, profoundly toxic, and can cause respiratory irritation or pulmonary hemorrhage.

226. (b). Oxford Miniature Vaporizer
The Oxford Miniature Vaporizer is a stainless steel, variable-bypass, draw-over vaporizer, flow over with wicks, non temperature compensated, multi agent.

227. (d). Boyle's ether bottle
The Boyle's bottle is a flow over vaporizer without wicks, if used with the plunger raised. When the vaporizer is on the highest mark and the plunger is depressed, the Boyle's ether bottle functions as a bubble through vaporizer. The cowl descends below the level of liquid ether and the surface area of the gas exposed to the liquid is maximized. The output is maximum when used in this way, though it rapidly falls as heat is lost from the system.

228. (a). Prevent misfilling
The filling systems are designed to prevent misfilling as modern vaporizers are designed to deliver accurate amounts of agent in the vapor form, taking into consideration their SVP. Misfilling will result in delivery of a mixture, the outcome of which is difficult to predict. Use of a more volatile agent results in an overdose.

229. (d). Keyed filling systems

230. (c). End tidal agent monitoring is not desirable

Titration of the syringe pump infusion rate will depend upon the monitoring of end-tidal volatile agent concentration and hemodynamic parameters. The Mirus incorporates automatic control of end-tidal concentrations.

231. (c). The same filter can be used as long as the patient is ventilated

The AnaConDa is intended for single use only and needs to be replaced every 24 hours or when needed.

232. (b). Performance is not significantly altered by changes in ambient pressure

The vapor output in terms of partial pressure varies very little with changes in ambient pressure. Since, the clinical effect depends upon the alveolar and brain partial pressure, no adjustment is required.

Temperature compensation is essential to compensate for the loss of latent heat of vaporization. The splitting ratio of the vaporizer is determined mainly by the saturated vapor pressure of the agent. Wicks increase the surface area available vaporization and ensure the presence of saturated vapor in the vaporization chamber.

233. (c). This is an electronic variable bypass vaporizer

The system is electronically monitored. Temperature compensation for loss of latent heat of vaporization is by supplied heat. High volatility (high SVP) and low potency (high MAC) are factors which make it unsuitable for delivery through mechanical variable bypass vaporizers.

234. (a). It can be filled while in use

They can be filled while in use, provided the dial setting is below 8% and flows are below 8 L/min.

They deliver the same output in v/v%, but, as ambient pressure falls this is a smaller fraction of the total pressure. Hence, the output in partial pressure (mmHg) falls.

They have been specifically designed to deliver desflurane as it is highly volatile and difficult to deliver through mechanical variable bypass vaporizers.

They do not have wicks. The sump is heated and pressurized and contains desflurane vapor when the vaporizer is operational.

235. (c). Audio visual alarms

The mechanical vaporizers do not have audio visual alarm systems as seen in the electronically regulated systems.

Fraser Sweatman developed the pin-index (color coding) and selectatec systems (vaporizer exclusion systems) are safety features of Ohio vaporizers.

236. (b). Vaporizer exclusion systems

Only one Aladin cassette can be slotted into place at a time and the cassettes are recognized by the magnets on the cassettes, so vaporizer exclusion systems are redundant in this design.

237. (d). Total fresh gas flow must increase to increase vaporizer output

The advantage of injection vaporizers over variable by pass vaporizers is that the vaporizer output is delinked from the fresh gas flow and can be independently increased. This prevents wastage and theatre pollution.

238. (d). Vaporizer in circuit location

They are plenum vaporizers placed on the back bar, located out of circuit.

239. (d). Concentration control dial

Leaks may be obvious – smell of agent, or insiduous – falling agent concentration and expired tidal volumes. Vaporizer filling ports and vaporizer machine interface are the most likely sites of improper seals.

240. (a). Mechanical variable bypass vaporizers

241. (b). Is reduced with the transfusion of red cells that were >14 days old

Koch et al. compared 2,872 patients who received red cells that were <14 days old with 3,130 patients who received red cells that were >14 days old, in a retrospective study of cardiac surgical patients in 2008. The risk of postoperative complications was shown to be significantly increased and short and long-term survival were shown to be reduced when transfused with older red cells, after adjusting for patient factors and surgical details.

242. (d). Cancer recurrence

Blood transfusion has been shown to have immunomodulatory effects. These may be associated with better outcomes after renal, cardiac, and liver transplantation. The outcome is worse in cancer recurrence, perioperative infection, and metastasis.

243. (c). Liver transplantation

Blood transfusion has been shown to have immunomodulatory effects. These may be associated with better outcomes after renal, cardiac, and liver transplantation. The outcome is worse in cancer recurrence, perioperative infection, and metastasis.

244. (b). A post-transfusion to pre-transfusion brain natriuretic peptide ratio of >1.5

TACO may be an extremely under-reported complication. It occurs either during massive transfusion or during too rapid transfusion.

Acute heart failure, is indicated by chest X-ray showing interstitial edema, possibly in association with cardiomegaly. A post-transfusion to pre-transfusion brain natriuretic peptide ratio of >1.5, if available, is diagnostic.

245. **(d). AB is the universal recipient type**
The term 'fresh frozen plasma' is confusing as plasma cannot be fresh and frozen at the same time. Fresh refers to time from collection, which is typically within eight hours of collection. The word frozen refers to the long-term storage condition. FFP transfusion must be ABO compatible. Blood group AB is the universal donor for plasma, as the plasma of type AB individuals lacks both anti-A and anti-B antibodies.

However, there is chronic shortage of this blood type as only 4% individuals are AB.

246. **(d). Deficient in fibrinogen**
FFP is sourced from either single units of whole blood (approximately 250 mL) or plasma collected by apheresis from donors (usually 500 mL). It is collected in citrate-containing solution, frozen within 8 hours of collection and can be stored at -30°C for up to 1 year. FFP contains fibrinogen (400–900 mg/unit).

247. **(d). There are no added anticoagulants**
FFP contains all of the clotting factors, fibrinogen (400–900 mg/unit), plasma proteins (particularly albumin), electrolytes, physiological anticoagulants (protein C, protein S, antithrombin, tissue factor pathway inhibitor) and added anticoagulants (citrate-containing anticoagulant solution)

248. **(d). Active bleeding and an International Normalized Ratio (INR) greater than 1.5**
Plasma transfusion is recommended in patients with active bleeding and an INR greater than 1.5, or before an invasive procedure or surgery if a patient has been anticoagulated.

249. **(d). In the ABO system, Type AB individuals have circulating plasma anti-A and anti-B antibodies**
In the ABO system, Type A individuals have circulating plasma anti-B antibodies, Type B have anti-A antibodies, Type O has both, and Type AB has neither.

250. **(c). This does not ultimately progress to cirrhosis, cardiomyopathy, diabetes, arthritis, and testicular failure**
Each unit of red blood cells contains 250 mg of iron. In the absence of an excretion mechanism, repeated transfusions result in iron accumulation in tissues which may ultimately lead progress to organa failure as mentioned above.

251. **(d). The risk with red cell concentrates is the highest**
The major bacterial contaminants are skin organisms acquired at the time of donation. Two strategies have been highly effective in reducing bacterial contamination - improved decontamination of puncture site with chlorhexidine in alcohol and discarding the initial flow of blood before it enters the collection bag. Platelets have the highest risk of bacterial contamination (1:2000) because they are stored at room temperature. The risk with red cell concentrates is much lower at 1:500 000.

252. **(a). More common with increasing age**
There are several near misses, for every incorrect blood component transfused. The risk is greater in children, commonly due to the failure of identity checks before transfusion. Also, transfusion is less common in children and staff may be less familiar with the associated hazards.
Anesthetized patients are at high risk as they are unable to confirm their identity details and access to bracelets may be difficult during surgery.

253. **(a). Leucodepletion has no effect on viral transmission**
Viral contamination of blood is now extremely rare because of leucodepletion, the suspension of red cells in minimal amounts of plasma, and careful donor selection.
Donated blood is routinely screened for human immunodeficiency virus (HIV), hepatitis B and C, and human T cell lymphoma virus 1. Leucodepletion has greatly reduced the transmission of cytomegalovirus (CMV); however, blood is still screened for specific vulnerable groups of recipients such as fetuses, neonates, and pregnant women receiving elective transfusions.

254. **(c). Decrease in potassium**
There is a reduction in ATP, 2,3-diphosphoglycerate and increase in lactate in stored packed cells. This results in fall in pH which leads to cell membrane rigidity and cell lysis. Thus, releasing the intracellular potassium resulting in increase potassium ions as the duration of storage increases.

255. **(b). Bacterial**
Though the risk of transfusion related transmission of viral diseases has diminished, the risk of bacterial transmission persists. The occurence of sepsis and the morbidity and mortality would depend on the number of transfusions and the underlying condition of the patient.

256. **(b). Platelets**
Bacterial contamination is more likely with platelet concentrates than when red cells are used and is the least in plasma. This is because platelets are stored at room temperature.

257. **(d). Pooled platelet concentrates from buffy coats have a lower bacterial contamination rate compared to apheresis platelets.**

Pooled platelet concentrates from buffy coats have a higher bacterial contamination rate compared to apheresis platelets. There is a 5.4 fold increased rate of septic transfusion reaction with pooled-donor platelets.

258. **(d). Asymptomatic individuals with past history of covid infection (antibody positive) should be barred from blood donation**
The FDA recommends that individuals who are tested and found positive for SARS-CoV-2 antibodies, but who did not have prior diagnostic testing and never developed symptoms, can donate without a waiting period and without performing a diagnostic test (e.g., nasopharyngeal swab),

259. **(a). Individuals who received a COVID-19 vaccine cannot donate blood**
The FDA recommends that vaccinated individuals can donate blood with the aforementioned caveats

260. **(c). Individuals diagnosed with COVID-19 or who are suspected of having COVID-19, and who had symptomatic disease, need not refrain from donating blood**
The FDA recommends that individuals diagnosed with COVID-19 or who are suspected of having COVID-19, and who had symptomatic disease, refrain from donating blood for at least 14 days after complete resolution of symptoms.

261. **(d). Tetralogy of Fallot**
IV induction will be faster in a patient with a right-to-left intracardiac shunt.
Tetralogy of Fallot is a cyanotic heart defect characterized by a ventricular septal defect (VSD), overriding aorta, right ventricular hypertrophy, and right ventricular outlet obstruction, which results in right-to-left shunting through the VSD.

262. **(a). Spread of local anesthetic to the femoral nerve**
Inadvertent femoral nerve block is a known complication of ilioinguinal and iliohypogastric nerve blocks. It happens due to local anesthetic spread along the fascia iliaca, below the inguinal ligament.

263. **(c). Decreases alveolar surface tension**
Surfactant lowers alveolar surface tension, prevents end-expiratory atelectasis, maintains functional residual capacity (FRC), resulting in improved lung compliance.

264. **(b). Controlled rapid sequence induction and intubation with cuffed ETT**
'Classic' RSII was described as 'preoxygenation / intravenous barbiturate/cricoid pressure/muscle relaxant/ rapid intubation' technique Cricoid pressure reduces LES, tone and with no information on the extent of force required to occlude the upper esophagus in children, excess force can distort airway making intubation more difficult. 'Controlled' RSII technique (cRSII) with gentle facemask ventilation (pressure <10–12 cm H_2O) prior to intubation is a safer and more appropriate approach in pediatric patients. With availability of cuffed ETT for pediatric patients, this is the best plan.

265. **(c). It is more common in males and more often found on the left side**

266. **(d). Will always require re-intubation**

267. **(a). URTI >4 weeks ago**

268. **(b). Broncho-pulmonary dysplasia**

269. **(d). Metabolic alkalosis**
Persistent vomiting in CHPS leads to loss of sodium, potassium, chloride, and hydrogen ions, causing hypochloremic metabolic alkalosis.

270. **(a). Take him to the or, consider it emergent, rapid-sequence induction and intubation (RSII)**
Children with suspected torsion of testis require immediate investigations and surgery to preserve potentially viable testis. They are assumed to have a full stomach and should have a RSII.

271. **(c). Desaturation and apnea**
Subarachnoid and epidural blockade in infants and small children is characterized by hemodynamic stability, even when the level of block is extensive. They rely more on the diaphragm for maintaining tidal volumes; thus, desaturation and apnea may be the first sign of total spinal.

272. **(b). Using MR-safe monitors**
Radiofrequency (RF) fields used by the MR scanner can cause thermal injury, especially coiled loops of cables (if not MR safe) contacting the patient's body.

273. **(b). 15 Years female undergoing squint surgery with h/o motion sickness**
Incidence of PONV is high in squint surgery, specially in adolescent girls with H/O motion sickness.

274. **(c). Glottic opening as the narrowest part of airway, with elliptical cross-section**
It is a myth that pediatric larynx is funnel (conical)-shaped with the narrowest area being the cricoid region which is circular in cross-section.

275. **(b). Heavy sedation since these kids are aggressive**
The prevalence of obstructive sleep apnea (OSA) in the pediatric population with Down syndrome is reported to be 45–76%. These kids are non-combative and hence heavy sedation in them is dangerous.

276. **(b). Congenital diaphragmatic hernia**
Positive pressure ventilation with face mask will lead to inflation of stomach which is occupying thoracic cavity in CDH. This will decompensate the neonate.

277. **(d). 0.5 mg/kg, ≤20 mg**

278. **(d). Prophylactic intravenous steroids**

279. **(c). Highest till 2 years of age**

280. **(b). ST segment, T wave amplitude changes**

281. **(b). Neck circumference > 42 cm**

282. **(d). Laryngoscopic response is reduced**

283. **(a). Intermittent pneumatic calf compression**

284. **(a). Depth of anesthesia monitoring and neuromuscular block monitoring**
Depth of anesthesia monitoring is essential in bariatric anesthesia, due to the rapid redistribution of IV anesthetic agents.
- To prevent awareness under general anesthesia immediately after induction
- To prevent oversedation
- To minimize residual sedation.

Neuromuscular block monitoring to prevent incomplete neuromuscular block antagonism.

285. **(b). Dosing should be based upon lean body weight and titrated to effect**
Lean body weight reflects excess non-adipose tissue of obese patients. This can be considerably greater than ideal body weight, generally peaking at 100 kg and 70 kg for male and female patients, respectively. Most of the drugs are given based on lean body weight, exceptions are noradrenaline and adrenaline are dosed according to ideal body weight and suxamethonium according to total body weight.

286. **(d). Good preoperative optimization of comorbidities and compliance**

287. **(d). Treated and optimized obstructive sleep apnea**

288. **(b). Bag-mask ventilation with PEEP before endotracheal intubation**
BMV with PEEP would cause gastric distension, splinting of diaphragm and further reduction in FRC before intubation, leading to desaturation.

289. **(d). METs > 4, OSA/OHS effectively treated by NIV and able to continue VTE prophylaxis at home if required**

290. **(b). Evidence of hypoventilation and desaturation if not stimulated**

291. **(c) 53%**
- ppoFEV1% = preoperative FEV1% X (1- % functional lung tissue removed/100)
- The left lung has 20 subsegments (10 in upper lobe and 10 in the lower lobe) whereas the right lung has 22 subsegments (6 in upper lobe, 4 in the middle lobe and 12 in the lower lobe)
- Hence after a left lower lobectomy a patient with a preoperative FEV_1 of 70% of normal would be expected to have a postoperative FEV_1 = 70% × (1 − 23.8/100) = 53.34%
- Hence % of functional lung tissue removed after left lower lobectomy = 10/42 × 100 = 23.8
- Therefore, after a left lower lobectomy a patient with a preoperative FEV_1 of 70% of normal would be expected to have a postoperative FEV_1 = 70% × (1 − 23.8/100) = 53.34%.

292. **(b). Cardiac output monitoring**
The ECOM-DLT (ECOM Medical, Inc., San Juan Capistrano, CA) contains multiple electrodes on the cuff and the tube that continuously measure the bioimpedance signal from the ascending aorta, in close proximity to the trachea. This device when connected to the ECOM monitor, in conjunction with an arterial catheter, provides cardiac output measurements.

293. **(a). Ileum**
The ileum is the final section of the small intestine. It absorbs vitamin B12 and other products of digestion that were not previously absorbed in the jejunum.

294. **(c). Interstitial cells of Cajal**
The myenteric plexus controls motility, which is carried out by enteric neurons, interstitial cells of Cajal (pacemaker cells that generate intrinsic electrical activity of the GI tract).
Notable cell types in the stomach that aid in digestion are:
- Mucous cells- protect against harsh hydrochloric acid
- Parietal cells which secrete hydrochloric acidb
- Chief cells which secrete pepsin and
- G cells those secrete gastrin.

Together these cells' secretions break down and partially digest the food into chyme as well as reduce particle dimension to an appropriate size (2 mm or less) before it enters the small intestine.
Paneth cells are specialized secretory epithelial cells that are located in the small intestinal crypts and produce a diverse group of antimicrobial, immune system-stimulating and trophic molecules.

295. **(b). Patient on a high dose of noradrenaline**
Drug-induced delayed gastric emptying edconditions include the administration of opioids and the use of vasoactive agents. Vasoactive drugs increase catecholamine concentrations leading to sympathetic stimulation and, therefore, decreased motility. These drugs are

often given intraoperatively or to critically ill patients for blood pressure control. Neurologic disorders resulting in decreased gastric motility include vagal neuropathies and gastroparesis. Hperglycemia, increased intracranial pressure, and mechanical ventilation can decrease gastric motility. Efforts to increase motility using drugs like erythromycin and metoclopramide have been used with some success.

296. (a). **Effect of nitrous oxide on perioperative cardiovascular events and mortality in patients undergoing major non cardiac surgery**
Study showed that nitrous oxide did not increase the risk of death and cardiovascular complications or surgical-site infection

297. (d). **Uterus**
Pain originating in the liver, pancreas, diaphragm, spleen, stomach, small bowel, ascending and proximal transverse colon, adrenal glands, kidneys, aorta, and mesentery passes through the celiac plexus, and is further transmitted via the thoracic splanchnic nerves to the central nervous system.

298. (a). **Vasoactive intestinal polypeptide**

299. (a). **Dramatic fall in BP**

300. (c). **Shunt**
The effect of a moderate shunt can be reduced, but not eliminated, by giving more oxygen because the non-ventilated region cannot be reached by the inspired gas. Thus, shunt will always lower PaO_2 at any PIO_2, as compared with what would have been measured without shunt. When the shunt increases to 25%, the rise in PaO_2 will be small, and with a shunt of 30% or greater, almost no effect of added O_2 can be seen. This is the net effect of mixing blood with normal pulmonary end-capillary PO_2 and shunt blood with mixed venous PO_2. If the latter is a large enough fraction of total lung blood flow, the additional O_2 that can be physically dissolved by the raised PIO_2 is so small that it is almost immeasurable. The shunt is said to be refractory.

301. (a). **Zone 1**

302. (d). **Emphysema**
Regions with low V/Q are caused by airway and vascular narrowing. This reduces ventilation and blood flow in some regions and increases them in others. Examples are obstructive lung disease and vascular disorders. Asthma, bronchitis, and emphysema do not cause a shunt. If a shunt is found, it indicates a complication.
Shunt is caused by the complete cessation of ventilation in a region, usually as a result of collapse or consolidation (pneumonia, edema, obliterative processes).

303. (b). **Increasing LV thickness**
Laplace's law states that wall stress (σ) is the product of pressure (P) and radius (R) divided by wall thickness (h)5: $\sigma = P \times R/2h$
In aortic stenosis, afterload is increased. The ventricle generates higher pressure to overcome the increased load opposing systolic ejection of blood. To generate such high pressure, the ventricle increases its wall thickness leading to left ventricular hypertrophy. By applying Laplace's law, increased left ventricular wall thickness will decrease wall stress, despite the increase in left ventricular pressure to overcome the aortic stenosis.

304. (c). **12 mL/kg**

305. (d). **Residual volume**

306. (b). **2%**

307. (c). **Dantrolene has a half-life of 10 hours**

308. (d). **72 hours**

309. (c). **ASA physical status was not found as a risk factor for AAGA**
- The estimated incidence of awareness is approximately 1:19,000 anesthetics. However, this incidence varied considerably in different settings.
- AAGA occurred most commonly the period from the start of induction of anesthesia to the start of the surgical intervention.
- Factors increasing the risk of accidental awareness included: female sex, age (younger adults, but not children), obesity, anaesthetist seniority (junior trainees), previous awareness, out-of-hours operating, emergencies, type of surgery (obstetric, cardiac, thoracic), and use of neuromuscular blocking agent.
- ASA physical status, race, and use or omission of nitrous oxide were not at risk for developing AAGA.

310. (d). **Tachycardia in response to increased right atrial filling pressures**

311. (d). **0.01 mg/kg**

312. (d). **For a reliable isoelectric EEG, the interelectrode impedances should be less than 10,000 ohms but more than 100 ohms**
- The usual base frequency in an awake patient is the beta range (>13 Hz).
- Deep sleep and anesthesia generally exhibit alpha frequency signals (8 to 13 Hz) on EEG.
- The EEG is produced by a summation of excitatory and inhibitory postsynaptic potentials produced in cortical gray matter.
- Electrocerebral silence (isoelectric EEg) is defined as no electroencephalographic activity above

2 µV/mm when recording from scalp electrode pairs placed 10 or more cm apart and with interelectrode impedances less than 10,000 ohms but more than 100 ohms.

313. **(c). Adding PEEP during mechanical ventilation decreases the cyclical shear stress injury**
    - Earlier in mid 1970s, the target of treatment in ARDS was to maintain normal arterial PCO_2 (with tidal volumes 10–12 mL/kg and PO_2 and normal PO_2 using FiO_2 and PEEP. The concept of baby lung brought a change in the goal of ARDS therapy from maintaining normal gas exchange to protective lung treatment using low tidal volumes while maintaining adequate oxygenation and accepting high PCO_2.
    - AECC ARDS definition was refined 2012 with the Berlin definition. Berlin definition removed the use of PCWP to rule out cardiogenic edema and it acknowledged the fact that heart failure and ARDS can coexist in the same patient.
    - Addition of PEEP can reduce VILI by increasing the resting end expiratory lung volume in the recruitable lung. Hence it avoids atelectrauma by preventing its cyclical collapse.

314. **(c). Total airway obstruction and death after tracheal extubation due to blood clot following nasal surgery**

315. **(d). Merocel laser guard has been FDA approved to wrap the endotracheal tubes during laser surgery**
    - Like oxygen, nitrous oxide is also a powerful oxidizer. Therefore adds to the risk of airway fires during laser surgery.
    - Laser Shield II is a silicone-based tube that is smoothly wrapped by a coated aluminum tape.
    - The Laser Flex tube (Mallinckrodt Inc, St. Louis, MO) is an airtight stainless steel spiral with two distal, saline-inflatable PVC cuffs (redundant in case of puncture of the proximal cuff).
    The Bivona Fome-Cuf (Smith's Medical, Kent, UK) is an aluminum spiral tube with self-inflating foam sponge-filled cuff.
    - The Merocel Laser Guard (Medtronic Xomed Merocel Corp, Mystic, CT) is a commercial, FDA-approved endotracheal wrap consisting of an adhesive metal foil laminated to a synthetic sponge surface. The manufacturer recommends this product only for use with CO_2 lasers. Laser Guard can be applied only to the shaft of the tube and provides no protection for the cuff.

316. **(c). Unlike sodalime, Lithium hydroxide-based absorbers do not need an additional catalyst**
    - Baralyme is a mixture of 80% calcium hydroxide and 20% barium hydroxide
    - The amount of CO generated at equipotent anesthetic concentrations for the different volatile agents is generally described as: desflurane ≥ enflurane > isoflurane ≥ halothane ≥ sevoflurane

317. **(d). i-gel**
    When LMA is used during MRI, the ferrous content in the pilot valve interferes with the MRI findings, and this may sometimes lead to a misdiagnosis. An in-vitro study of six SGAs (Classic, Unique, ProSeal, Supreme, Ambu AuraOnce, i-gel) showed artifacts in all except two devices Ambu and i-gel (no ferrous content) suggesting their suitability for MRI. The other available MRI compatible devices are AES Ultra, Solus™ LMA (Intersurgical, Berkshire, UK) and Laryseal™ MRI (Flexicare Medical Ltd., MG, UK).

318. **(d). Radiation**

319. **(a). Using recruitment methods and PEEP to open the collapsed alveolar units**

320. **(a). It is calculated as peak airway pressure minus PEEP in patients who are mechanically ventilated without any spontaneous efforts**
    Driving pressure (ΔP) is calculated as the difference between plateau pressure (P_{plat}) and positive end-expiratory pressure (PEEP).

321. **(b). Berlin definition**

322. **(a). Petechial rash**
    Chonfeld Fat Embolism Syndrome Index
    - 5 points: petechial rash
    - 4 points: diffuse alveolar infiltrates
    - 3 points: hypoxemia (PaO_2 < 70 mm Hg with an FiO_2 1)
    - 1 point: confusion, fever, tachycardia, tachypnea.
    5 or more points are needed to make a diagnosis.

323. **(d). Phase IV or V**
    Korotkoff measured blood pressure by auscultating sounds generated by arterial blood flow. These sounds are a complex series of audible frequencies produced by turbulent flow beyond the partially occluding cuff. The pressure at which the first Korotkoff sound is heard is generally accepted as systolic pressure (phase I). The character of the sound progressively changes (phases II and III), becomes muffled (phase IV), and is finally absent (phase V). Diastolic pressure is recorded at phase IV or V. However, phase V may never occur in certain pathophysiologic states such as aortic regurgitation.

324. **(c). Disappearance of radial pulse by palpation during cuff inflation**

325. **(d). Higher systolic and lower diastolic pressure**

326. **(a). Exaggerated inspiratory fall in systolic arterial pressure during quiet breathing**

327. **(b). Severe ventricular systolic dysfunction**
    Pulsus alterans (alternate strong and weak beat) is found in severe ventricular dysfunction. It is usually usually associated with an S3 gallop, which signifies advanced myocardial disease, and often disappears with treatment of heart failure.

328. **(a). Urinary sodium levels are generally <20 mEq/L**
    - In SIADH, urinary sodium levels are generally >40 mEq/L.
    - In hypovolemic hyponatremia they are <20 mEq/L.

329. **(d). The terminal portion of the motor neurone is unmyelinated**
    - The synaptic cleft is 20 nanometres wide
    - The Depths of the folds repopulated with Sodium channels while the shoulders are densely populated with acetylcholine receptors
    - A single muscle fiber is innervated by a single branch of a motor neurone – together they are termed a motor unit. Although a single motor neurone may send branches to a number of muscle fibers, each muscle fiber receives input from only one nerve.

330. **(b). The ligamentum flavum connects the adjacent laminae**
    - The anterior longitudinal ligament travels along the anterior aspect of the vertebral bodies. While the posterior longitudinal ligament travels along the posterior aspect of the vertebral bodies and therefore at the anterior aspect of the vertebral foramen.
    - The interspinous ligaments connect adjacent spinous processes with no connection between adjacent ligaments. Supraspinous ligament is a tough fibrous ligament running along the tips of the spinous processes from C7 down to the sacrum. It can become ossified in the elderly.
    - The ligamentum flava are elastic ligaments, they provide much of the natural recoil of the spine.

331. **(b). The osmoreceptors that sense osmolality of body fluids are located in posterior hypothalamus**
    Osmolality acts via osmoreceptors, receptors that sense the osmolality of the body fluids. These osmoreceptors are located in the anterior hypothalamus.

332. **(a). Posterior cerebral artery is a branch of the internal carotid artery**
    The intracranial parts of the vertebral arteries unite at the caudal border of the pons to form the basilar artery. The vertebrobasilar arterial system and its branches are often referred to clinically as the posterior circulation of the brain. The Basilar artery ends by dividing into the two posterior cerebral arteries.

333. **(c). Lateral pterygoid**
    - MTM (Masseter, Temporalis, Medial pterygoid) are elevators of mandible, to close the mouth.
    - Lateral pterygoid is depressor of mandible to open the mouth.

334. **(b). Suprahyoid**

335. **(c). Tympanomandibular**
    TM joint has a capsular ligament strengthened by temporomandibular, sphenomandibular, and stylomandibular ligaments.

336. **(a). Primary curves are concave forward**
    Vertebral column has four curvatures that occur in the cervical, thoracic, lumbar, and sacral regions. The fetal thoracic and sacral kyphoses are concave anteriorly, whereas the acquired cervical and lumbar lordoses are concave posteriorly.
    The cervical lordosis becomes evident when an infant begins to raise (extend) the head while prone and to hold the head erect while sitting.
    The lumbar lordosis becomes apparent when the child learns to assume the upright posture for standing and walking

337. **(c). Phrenic nerve**
    - The pain due to pericarditis originates in the parietal layer only and is transmitted by the phrenic nerve.
    - The fibrous pericardium and parietal layer of serous pericardium are supplied by the phrenic nerve. Visceral layer of serous pericardium is insensitive to pain.

338. **(a). The central chemoreceptors are located near the dorsal surface of the pons**
    The central chemoreceptors are located near the ventral surface of the medulla. These chemoreceptors have an important role in responding to changes in the arterial tension of CO_2, but not oxygen as would be expected.
    The central chemoreceptors are surrounded by extracellular fluid of the brain, which is in contact with the cerebrospinal fluid (CSF). The pH of cerebrospinal fluid is slightly acidic compared with plasma because it contains fewer proteins and hence a lesser ability to buffer pH changes.
    The changes in pH in the CSF caused by the increased CO_2 are exaggerated when compared with plasma, because of its limited buffering capacity. Respiratory acidosis causes a greater increase in ventilation than metabolic acidosis simply because the blood–brain

barrier is permeable to CO_2. Patients who are chronic CO_2 retainers have a compensated near-normal CSF pH, so ventilation is comparatively low for the level of CO_2. These patients rely on their hypoxic drive (and hence the peripheral chemoreceptors) for ventilation.

339. **(b). The intercostal nerves run between the internal intercostal muscle and the transversus thoracic muscle**
    - The intercostal nerves are formed from the ventral primary rami of the spinal nerves of T1–T11. The dorsal primary rami supply the skin over the spine.
    - Both rami contain sensory, motor and autonomic fibers and can be anaesthetised by a paravertebral block.
    - The intercostal nerves run between the internal and the innermost intercostal muscles at the superior end of the intercostal space.

340. **(b). 85% of the cranial volume is occupied by brain parenchyma**
    A: The mass of the adult human brain is 1400 g.
    B and C: Total volume of CSF is 150 mL but 75 mL is in the spinal intrathecal space so only 75–100 mL is in the cranial vault. This represents 7–10% of the intracranial volume. Between 5% and 8% is the cerebral blood volume, leaving 85% of the intracranial volume occupied by brain parenchyma.
    Early compensation mechanisms for rising ICP include displacement and reabsorption of CSF, but not reduced production.

341. **(b). The internal jugular vein begins at the foramen lacerum at the base of the skull**
    - The internal jugular vein is the largest vein in the neck and represents the continuation of the sigmoid sinus at the jugular foramen. It drains the brain and superficial areas of the head and neck
    - Behind the sternal end of the clavicle the vein unites with the subclavian vein to form the brachiocephalic vein. Near its termination, the inferior bulb of the internal jugular vein is noted, and this contains a bicuspid valve.

342. **(a). Blood-nerve barrier is formed by the endoneurium**
    - Within a nerve, each axon is surrounded by a layer of connective tissue called the endoneurium.
    - The axons are bundled together into groups called fascicles, and each fascicle is wrapped in a layer of connective tissue called the perineurium. It is this perineurium that forms the blood–nerve barrier and therefore acts as a diffusion barrier to local anesthetics.

343. **(c). Conduction velocity of Aα fibers is 70–120 m/second**

344. **(b). Sacral hiatus is formed by inferior articular process of S5**
    - The sacral vertebral foramina form a triangular canal called the sacral canal, which is a continuation of the lumbar spinal canal.
    - Sacral hiatus is formed by failure of the laminae of S5 to meet, thus exposing its dorsal surface. Sacral cornuae are formed by inferior articular process of S5 of each side.
    - Practically, the sacral hiatus is identified by drawing an equilateral triangle, the base of which is formed by the posterior superior iliac spine.

345. **(b). The right celiac ganglion is slightly lower than the left ganglion**
    - The celiac plexus is located anterior to the aorta at the level of the L1 vertebral body and anterior to the crura of the diaphragm.
    - This plexus contains grossly two large discrete ganglia on either side of the aorta. The left celiac ganglion is slightly lower than the right ganglion.

346. **(d). Bronchogenic cyst**
    - Bronchogenic cyst (foregut structures) arises from middle mediastinum.

347. **(d). RCA supplies to the right bundle branch**
    - Right coronary artery has smaller lumen as compared with left coronary artery (left ventricle is thicker than right).
    - The right coronary artery arises from the anterior aortic sinus, supplies major portion of right atrium and ventricle.
    - Circumflex artery is a branch of left coronary artery and is the exclusive supply to the right bundle branch.

348. **(a). Posterior interventricular artery**
    - Coronary dominance is determined by posterior interventricular artery (PIVA).
    - In about 65% of the population PIVA is given by right coronary artery alone (right cardiac dominance), in 10% cases it is a branch of left coronary artery alone (left cardiac dominance) and in the remaining 25 % it is given by both (balanced dominance).

349. **(c). Pressure work**
    - Pressure work uses most of the oxygen, 65%, followed by basal requirements = 20%, volume work = 15%, with only 1% of the supplied oxygen being used for electrical activity.

350. **(c). Glossopharyngeal nerve**

351. **(b). C3–C6**

352. **(d). New alveoli continue to develop until 2 years of age**

New alveoli continue to develop until about age 8 years, by which time there are approximately 300 million alveoli.

353. **(c). The opening of the coronary sinus lies between the IVC orifice and the SVC orifice**
    - The interior of the right atrium has a smooth, thin-walled, posterior part (the sinus venarum) on which the venae cavae (SVC and IVC) and coronary sinus open, bringing poorly oxygenated blood into the heart.
    - The opening of the coronary sinus, a short venous trunk receiving most of the cardiac veins, is between the right AV orifice and the IVC orifice.

354. **(c). Both the right and the left bundle branch of the AV bundle are supplied by the left coronary artery**
    - Both bundle branches of the conduction system of heart are located in anterior 2/3 of ventricular septum; which is supplied by branches of the left coronary artery.
    - The posterior 1/3 of the ventricular septum is supplied by the right coronary artery in right dominance and from the left coronary artery in left dominance. However, this is irrelevant to this question because the bundle branches of the conduction system of the heart lie approximately midway (from ventral to dorsal) in the ventricular septum, ie in the anterior 2/3 of the septum.

355. **(c). Posterior mediastinum contains the thoracic aorta, thoracic duct and lymphatic trunks**
    - The posterior mediastinum is located inferior to the transverse thoracic plane. It lies anterior to the T5–T12 vertebrae, posterior to the pericardium and diaphragm, and between the parietal pleura of the two lungs
    - The posterior mediastinum contains the thoracic aorta, thoracic duct and lymphatic trunks, posterior mediastinal lymph nodes, azygos and hemi-azygos veins, and esophagus and esophageal nerve plexus.

356. **(c). Phrenic nerves**
    - The posterior mediastinum contains the thoracic aorta, thoracic duct and lymphatic trunks, posterior mediastinal lymph nodes, azygos and hemi-azygos veins, and esophagus and esophageal nerve plexus.
    - Phrenic nerve is in middle mediastinum.

357. **(a). Cisterna chyli**

358. **(b). Vagus nerve**
    The esophageal hiatus is an oval opening for the esophagus in the muscle of the right crus of the diaphragm at the level of the T10 vertebra.
    The esophageal hiatus also transmits the anterior and posterior vagal trunks, esophageal branches of the left gastric vessels, and a few lymphatic vessels.

359. **(a). External intercostal muscle**
    Diaphragm and to some extent external intercostal muscles are used in quiet breathing. Internal intercostals, subcostals and abdominal muscles are used during forceful expiration.

360. **(c). In pulmonary embolism anatomical dead space increases**

361. **(c). CN IX**
    - Sensory supply of posterior one third of the tongue is by glossopharyngeal nerve.
    - Anterior two third of the tongue is supplied by (sensory supply) lingual nerve which is a branch of mandibular division of Trigeminal (Vth) nerve.
    - Hypoglossal nerve is the motor supply of the muscles of the tongue.

362. **(b). It lies superficial to sternocleidomastoid**
    It lies deep to the sternocleidomastoid muscle.

363. **(b). 100 mL/min**
    Uterine blood flow in non-pregnant state is 100 mL/min, and increases up to 700 mL/min, almost 10% of cardiac output at term.

364. **(b). 10% of cardiac output**

365. **(c). It is the most inferior of the three large diaphragmatic apertures**
    The most superior of the three large diaphragmatic apertures, the caval opening, lies at the level of the IV disc between the T8 and T9 vertebrae.
    During inspiration with contraction of diaphragm, the caval opening widens, which dilates the Inferior vena cava.

366. **(d) Pelvic splanchnic nerves**
    - The parasympathetic part of the autonomic innervation of the abdominal viscera consists of the following:
        - Anterior and posterior vagal trunks.
        - Pelvic splanchnic nerves.
        - Abdominal (para-aortic) autonomic plexuses and their extensions, the periarterial plexuses.
        - Intrinsic (enteric) parasympathetic ganglia, components of intrinsic enteric plexuses of the enteric nervous system.

367. **(d). Dominance of the coronary arterial system depends on which artery gives rise to the posterior descending artery**
    - The right coronary artery (RCA) arises from the right aortic sinus of the ascending aorta. Near its origin, the RCA in around 80% people gives off an ascending sino-atrial nodal branch, which supplies the SA node.

- The left coronary artery (LCA) arises from the left aortic sinus. LCA divides into two branches, the anterior IV branch (left anterior descending artery) and the circumflex branch.
- In approximately 15% of hearts, the LCA is dominant in that the posterior IV branch is a branch of the circumflex artery.

368. **(d). The cardiac plexus is formed by sympathetic fibers alone**

369. **(c). It does not drain the right arm**
     - Large lymphatic vessels enter large collecting vessels, called lymphatic trunks, which unite to form either the right lymphatic duct or the thoracic duct
     - The right lymphatic duct drains lymph from the body's right upper quadrant (right side of the head, neck, and thorax plus the right upper limb). At the root of the neck, it enters the junction of the right internal jugular and right subclavian veins, the right venous angle
     - The thoracic duct drains lymph from the remainder of the body. The lymphatic trunks draining the lower half of the body merge in the abdomen, sometimes forming a dilated collecting sac, the cisterna chyli. From this sac (if present), or from the merger of the trunks, the thoracic duct ascends through the aortic hiatus in the diaphragm and then through the thorax to enter the left venous angle (junction of left nternal jugular and left subclavian veins).

370. **(d). Right bundle branch**
     - Right bundle branch is present in that region of the interventricular septum, which is exclusively supplied by left coronary artery.
     - In majority of the population SA node and AV node are supplied by right coronary artery.
     - Major portion of bundle of His is supplied by left coronary artery, and partly supplied by right coronary artery.

371. **(a). 10–12 cm**

372. **(c). T4**

373. **(b). 4–6 cm^2**

374. **(c). 4–6 mL/kg actual body weight**

375. **(b). To facilitate surgical exposure**
     - BPF and lung hemorrhage are indications for lung separation but are uncommon indications.
     - Lung separation during surgery is instituted most commonly for facilitating lung collapse and by increasing shunt can worsen gas exchange

376. **(c). Left lower lobectomy**
     In left lower lobectomy, a left sided DLT may be acceptable.

377. **(d). Hypoxic Pulmonary Vasoconstriction is primarily responsible for reducing shunt during OLV**
     - Vasodilators attenuate HPV
     - Inhalational agents can be used during one lung ventilation. MAC values below 1 do not affect HPV significantly
     - High PEEP can attenuate HPV.

378. **(a). Positive pressure ventilation is better than normal spontaneous breathing**
     - Posterolateral thoracotomy does not cause flail segment as ribs are not excised.
     - Chest drain is beneficial in the management of pneumothorax.
     - Epidural analgesia may be useful but not mandatory for management of a flail chest.

379. **(c). EZ blocker**
     All other blockers have single cuff.

380. **(c). Heimlich valve can be used in place of an underwater seal**
     Heimlich valve is a one way which can be used in place of an underwater seal. It is more convenient in ambulatory patients.
     Rationale
     - Negative pressure should not be applied in the post-pneumonectomy cavity
     - Usually a single chest drain is adequate but sometimes 2 chest drains viz. apical and basal may be inserted in lung resection surgery
     - 2 bottle system is superior to one bottle system when large amount of liquid is to be drained.

381. **(a). Clinical practice guidelines for lung resection surgery commonly use the predicted postoperative forced vital capacity (PPO FVC) value to determine risk**
     Rationale
     - Clinical practice guidelines for lung resection surgery commonly use the predicted post operative forced expired volume in 1 second (PPO FEV1) value to determine risk
     - Diffusion capacity of lung for carbon monoxide is affected by the blood hemoglobin level and therefore DLCO values corrected for hemoglobin (DLCOc) are used for interpretation.

382. **(d). Total lung capacity is the most important value for the interpretation of a standard spirometry test.**
     FVC and FEV1 are the more important values in interpretation of a spirometry test. Moreover, residual volume and TLC may not be routinely measured in a standard PFT.

383. **(b). Right upper lobe bronchus**
384. **(c). Critical velocity is velocity above which flow of a fluid changes from turbulent to laminar**
385. **(d). Heidbrink valve is a type of APL valve**
    - The maximum pressure allowed by the APL valve in the circle system in modern machines is certainly higher than 35 cm H_2O and is usually 70 cm H_2O.
    - Fresh gases can be vented out depending on the position of the APL valve relative to the position of the unidirectional valves and fresh gas flow connection and the fresh gas flow rate.
    - Position of the APL valve between the patient and the inspiratory unidirectional valve can cause rebreathing of carbon dioxide in the exhaled gases and is therefore and unacceptable position.
386. **(b). Deposition of water droplets in the proximal airways is a common problem with ultrasonic nebulizers.**
    Ultrasonic nebulizers are highly efficient but there is a significant risk of excessive water delivery to the alveoli which can lead to impaired gas exchange and atelectasis.
387. **(d). Droplets of <0.5 μm vaporize and do not reach the airways**
    Droplets <0.5 μm may be carried out with expired gases.
388. **(a). Compliance thermometer**
389. **(b). Isoflurane > sevoflurane > desflurane > nitrous oxide**
    Potency is directly related to the solubility coefficient in oil i.e. agents with lower MAC values have higher solubility coefficients.
390. **(b). Charles law : Calculating oxygen content of a pressurized oxygen cylinder**
    Boyles law: Temperature remaining constant, pressure is directly proportional to the volume. Hence volume of oxygen at atmospheric pressure can be calculated based on the pressure in the oxygen cylinder and volume of the cylinder.
    Daltons law of partial pressures: Fink effect. Rapid diffusion of nitrous oxide increases the concentration of nitrous oxide in the alveolus thereby reducing the concentration and partial pressure of oxygen.
    Jet nebulizer uses pressurized gases passing through a nozzle to cause Venturi effect. This entrains liquid which is sprayed onto an anvil which makes droplets of the liquid.
    Avogadgro's hypothesis : Calculating amount of gas in a nitrous oxide cylinder.
391. **(a). A person of group O is a universal donor**
392. **(c). Lower chloride ion concentration**
    Extracellular fluid has a higher chloride ion concentration as compared to intracellular fluid.
393. **(c). The pH is directly proportional to the hydrogen ion concentration**
394. **(a). Metabolic alkalosis is seen with prolonged use of loop diuretics**
395. **(c). It is decreased by aminophylline**
    It is proposed that aminophylline, a methyl xanthine derivative, produces bronchodilatation by increasing cyclic AMP levels in the bronchial smooth muscle.
396. **(c). Barbiturates maybe used to treat hyperbilirubinemia.**
    Phenobarbital increases bilirubin clearance by liver. It enhances bilirubin-UDP-glucuronyl transferase activity. Whether the influence on bilirubin clearance is related to the effect on the enzyme is unknown.
397. **(b). Increase in urinary nitrogen excretion**
    Starvation causes an increase in urinary nitrogen excretion initially with increase in gluconeogenesis but with prolonged starvation, the rate of protein catabolism reduces as measured by decrease in urinary nitrogen (urea) excretion.
398. **(d). End-stage liver disease**
    Blood urea nitrogen is decreased in end-stage liver disease secondary to impaired metabolic activity of the liver.
399. **(c). Corticotropin**
    The anterior pituitary gland produces corticotropin, a 39-residue hormone that activates the adrenal cortex.
400. **(c). Taq DNA polymerase**
    Only a DNA polymerase is capable of making multiple copies of the DNA sequence. HRP (Horseradish peroxidase) is an enzyme that is used in ELISA and immunohistochemistry tests. Restriction enzymes are EcorI and EcorII.
401. **(c). Saponification number**
    The saponification number is defined as the weight of potassium hydroxide, in milligrams, needed to saponify 1 g of fat.
402. **(b). Phosphofructokinase-1**
    Phosphofructokinase-1 is a regulatory enzyme that plays a key role in glycolysis control. When the cell's ATP supply is reduced, its activity increases.
403. **(b). NADH and the ATP/ADP ratio**
    The key determinants of whether glucose is metabolized by aerobic or anaerobic glycolysis are NADH and the ATP/ADP ratio.

404. **(c). Carbamoyl phosphate**
The urea cycle is entered by carbamoyl phosphate, which acts as an active carbamoyl group donor.

405. **(d). Lipids**
Carbohydrates provide 4 calories per gram, protein provides 4 calories per gram, and fat provides 9 calories per gram.

406. **(d). All of these**

407. **(b). 1:20**
The acid-base mechanism is maintained by the following formula. Catalyzed by carbonic anhydrase, carbon dioxide (CO_2) reacts with water (H_2O) to form carbonic acid (H_2CO_3), which in turn rapidly dissociates to form a bicarbonate ion (HCO_3^-) and a hydrogen ion (H^+).
As calculated by the Henderson-Hasselbalch equation, in order to maintain a normal pH of 7.4 in the blood (whereby the pKa of carbonic acid is 6.1 at physiological temperature), a 20:1 bicarbonate to carbonic acid must constantly be maintained.

408. **(a). Stereoisomers**
- Anomers is an epimer at the hemiacetal/hemiketal carbon in a cyclic saccharide, an atom called the anomeric carbon.
- Optical isomers are two compounds which contain the same number and kinds of atoms, bonds and different spatial arrangements of the atoms, but which have non-superimposable mirror images.
- Epimers is a stereoisomer that differs in configuration at any single stereogenic center.

409. **(a). Sucrose**
The Benedict's test identifies reducing sugars, however other reducing substances also give a positive reaction. This includes all monosaccharides and many disaccharides, including lactose and maltose. Sucrose (combination of fructose and glucose) is a non-reducing sugar, which does not react with Benedict's reagent.

410. **(a). Polysaccharide**
Starch is a polysaccharide comprising glucose monomers joined in α 1,4 linkages.

411. **(b). D-Fructose**
Dextrose is a dextrorotary optical isomers of fructose.

412. **(a). Diabetes mellitus**
When blood glucose level increases above 180 mg/dL, (10 mmol/L) it is secreted in the urine; and, every 35 to 40 mmol/kg increment in urine osmolality increases the urine specific gravity by 0.001.

413. **(c). Cori's cycle**

414. **(d). Muscles and adipose tissue**

415. **(a). Glucagon**

416. **(b). Lactate from muscles to liver**

417. **(b). Brain**

418. **(c). Polysaccharides**

419. **(d). Gluconeogenesis**

420. **(b). Two**

421. **(a). Pyruvate kinase**

422. **(a). β-hydroxy butyrate**
Three intermediate products of fat metabolism are acetoacetic acid, acetone and Beta-hydroxybutyrate. Acetoacetic acid, acetone react with an alkaline solution of sodium nitroprusside to form a purple-colored complex. This method can detect above 1-5 mg/dL of acetoacetic acid and 10–20 mg/dL of acetone. Beta-hydroxybutyrate is not detected by this method as it does not contain a keto group.

423. **(a). Selective competitive inhibitor of HMG-CoA reductase**

424. **(c). Diabetes mellitus and starvation**

425. **(a). It occurs in the small intestine**

426. **(d). Kreb's cycle**
Kreb's cycle, also known as TCA cycle or Citric acid cycle involves both catabolism and anabolism.

427. **(b). Brain**

428. **(c). Each individual**

429. **(a). Glycogen**

430. **(c). Plasma calcium is low and inorganic phosphorous high**

431. **(d). Creatinine clearance**

432. **(d). Urine osmolality**
Creatinine clearance and inulin clearance are functions of glomerular filtration. Para-aminohippurate (PAH) clearance measures renal plasma flow.

433. **(b). Post-synaptic inhibitor transmitter**

434. **(c). Urea**

435. **(d). Glutamine formation**

436. **(c). Phenylalanine**
Essential amino acids are the amino acids which can not be synthesized by the organism fast enough to meet the demand, therefore must come drom diet.
Histidine, isoleucine, leucine, lysine, methionine, phenylalanine, threonine, tryptophan, and valine are the nine essential amino acids.

437. (a). G-6 phosphatase deficiency

438. (a). Hemolytic jaundice
Urobilinogen is the end product of conjugated bilirubin metabolism. Conjugated bilirubin passes through the bile ducts, where it is metabolized by normal intestinal bacteria to urobilinogen.
Normally, about 50% of the urobilinogen is excreted in the stool, and 50% is reabsorbed into the enterohepatic circulation. A small amount of absorbed urobilinogen, about 1 to 4 mg/day, will escape hepatic uptake and be excreted in the urine.

439. (d). Decreased serum alkaline phosphatase and increased serum LDH and ALT

440. (c). 1.0 gm/kg of body weight

441. (a). Hemolytic jaundice

442. (c). Liver

443. (b). Ischemic hepatitis
Synthesis of coagulation factors is affected as adequate hepatocytes may not be present in liver damage.

444. (b). Arachidonic acid

445. (b). Fatty acids uncouple oxidative phosphorylation

446. (a). Creatine kinase
Creatine kinase (CK) or creatine phosphokinase (CPK) exists as 3 isoenzymes. Each isoenzyme is a dimmer composed of two subunits (M or B or both). Elevation of CPK2 (MB) in serum is an early reliable diagnostic indication of myocardial infarction.

447. (b). Acetazolamide

448. (c). Erythrocytes

449. (a). It is often a vitamin

450. (c). 2
Administration of 2 drugs of different class are recommended if the patient has 1 or 2 risk factors for PONV.

451. (d). 1–2 loose stools/day
More than 3 loose stools per day is considered as a symptom of gut dysfunction

452. (b). It is effective for blood infection showing gram negative bacilli
Vancomycin is ineffective in gram negative organisms, used only for gram positive organisms.

453. (d). In case of multi-lumen catheter, one set per lumen should be collected

454. (b). 12 mL/kg
According to ASRA guidelines for LAST toxicity, the maximum dose of intralipid which can be administered as 12 mL/kg.

455. (d.) ACE inhibitors

456. (c). Increased hydrogen ions
Increased H^+ ions leads to acidosis which facilitates the release of oxygen thereby shifting ODC to right.

457. (c). 60 mm Hg

458. (c). Both depolarization and repolarization
The QT interval includes both ventricular depolarization and repolarization.

459. (c). IU/hr
Insulin is secreted in the portal venous system at a basal rate of 1 IU/hr.

460. (d). All of the above

461. (d). Mivacurium

462. (a). 16, 18, 18 G

463. (b). Flow is inversely proportional to the length of the catheter
Flow is directly proportional to the fourth power of radius, and inversely proportional to the length of the catheter.

464. (a). Predict postoperative pulmonary complications
ARISCAT score is used for prediction of postoperative pulmonary complications

465. (a). Cardiopulmonary exercise testing

466. (b). Anterior, middle and posterior

467. (a). 2.5% Lignocaine + 2.5% Prilocaine

468. (c). 30 Fr

469. (d). Decrease in blood pressure
The Pringle maneuver is associated with a decrease in cardiac output and an increase in mean blood pressure; the former effect is due to a decreased venous return secondary to portal clamping while the latter effect is linked to arterial vasoconstriction, both mesenteric and systemic. Systemic vasoconstriction is secondary to the decreased venous return.

470. (b). 2, 7, 9, 10

471. (a). Common peroneal nerve represents most common neuropathy (78%)

472. (a). Prothrombin time (PT) represents integrity of intrinsic and common pathways
Prothrombin time represents integrity of extrinsic and common pathways, which evaluates factors II, V, VII, X and fibrinogen concentrations.

473. (c). 10

474. (a). Atrial contraction

475. (c). L5–S1
476. (a). Fifth and fourth sacral vertebrae
477. (d). Watcha scale is a better predictor than PAED scale
478. (a). Dense deposit disease (DDD)
    - Dense deposit disease (DDD), recurrence is almost universal after transplantation.
    - Reported rates are 80–100%.
    - Focal segmental glomerulosclerosis—20–30% recurrence
    - Membranous glomerulonephritis—10–20% recurrence
    - Membranoproliferative glomerulonephritis—20–30% recurrence
    - IgA nephropathy—40–50% recurrence.
479. (d). Meperidine
    Meperidine is to be avoided because it can accumulate in renal failure and lead to respiratory depression.
    Non steroidal anti inflammatory drugs (NSAIDS) should be avoided as well.
    Fentanyl, paracetamol and hydrocodone can be safely given.
480. (b). Presence of doll's eye movement
    For certifying brain death, the following need to be evaluated:
    Presence of irreversible coma; and, the cessation of spontaneous respiration confirmed with apnea tests, absence of pupillary light reflexes, corneal reflexes, doll's eye movements, gag reflex, cough reflex (tracheal), eye movements on caloric testing bilaterally, absence of motor response in any cranial nerve distribution, and motor response on stimulation of face/limb/trunk.
481. (d). Hormone cocktail containing thyroxine, insulin, steroids and vasopressin may be required in some cases
    Ventilatory status—If a lung harvest is planned, the doner should receive protective lung ventilation consisting of smaller tidal volume (6 mL/kg/min), positive end-expiratory pressure (positive end-expiratory pressure of 4–8 cm of water) and a low FiO_2.
    Hypovolemia due to the trauma or more commonly diabetes insipidus (DI) is countered by vasopressin infusion which also helps in maintain the systemic vascular resistance.
    Electrolyte imbalances such as hypokalemia and low calcium and magnesium need continuous correction.
    Hypothermia may aggravate these deleterious effects and normothermia should be the target.
    A 'hormone cocktail' of IV thyroxine, insulin, vasopressin and steroids is usually reserved for the BDD with borderline organ functions with a prolonged waiting period or requiring high inotropic supports.
482. (c). Patients with primary liver tumors for liver transplant
    The Milan criteria is used in selecting patients with primary liver tumors who may benefit from liver transplant.
483. (d). Increase in stroke volume
484. (c). Increase cerebral metabolic rate ($CMRO_2$)

Interventions for management of inadequate cerebral perfusion pressure.	
Rechice brain water	• Mamiitol • Hypertonic saline • Furosemide • Dexamethasone to decrease (peritumoraL vasogenic) edema
Remove CSF/CSF reduction	• External ventricular drain (EVD) • Lumbar drain • Acetazolamide (CSF reduction)
Decrease CBV/ Decrease $CMRO_2$	• Head up Tilt • Avoid constriction at the neck • Avoid PEEP and excessive pressure • Metabolic suppression: propofol, barbiturate (decrease $CMRO_2$) • Mild to moderate hyperventilation
Elevate MAP (CPP = MAP – ICP)	• Adequate intravascular volume resuscitation • Vasopressor

CBV = cerebral blood volume: CSF = cerebrospinal fluid: MAP = mean arterial pressure

485. (c). Shortened QT interval
486. (d). Nitrous oxide
    The use of remifentanil also facilitates a smooth, hemodynamically stable extubation allowing rapid neurological assessment. It can be used in conjunction with propofol or volatile agents for maintenance of anesthesia.
    Nitrous oxide should be avoided in neuroanesthesia as it causes cerebral vasodilation with a resulting increase in cerebral blood flow (CBF) and ICP.
    Dexamethasone (4e8 mg on induction) has dual benefits in neuroanesthesia. It reduces the risk of PONV, as well as reducing cerebral edema associated with tumors.
    Dexmedetomidine is a highly selective alpha-2 adrenoreceptor agonist, with several advantages. A growing number of studies have demonstrated its potential usefulness in the reduction in postoperative pain scores, and perioperative opioid consumption following neurosurgery.
487. (d). Platypnea
    Clinical signs in patients with HPS are digital clubbing, cyanosis, and platypnea (dyspnea that is worse upon

moving from supine to upright position). This form of dyspnea is unique to HPS.

488. **(c). Patients with pulmonary artery hypertension benefit with single lung transplant**
Single lung transplant is technically simpler than bilateral transplant and makes the best use of a limited resource.
Single lung transplant may be an appropriate choice for patients with COPD and interstitial lung disease.
Patients with suppurative lung disease or severe pulmonary hypertension require bilateral transplant. Notwithstanding this distinction, bilateral lung transplant is increasingly preferred for all patients because of mounting evidence for an overall survival benefit.
In 2017, bilateral transplant accounted for 80% of all lung transplants.

489. **(b). Neohepatic phase**
Pre-anhepatic phase: From skin incision to clamping of the inferior vena cava (IVC), portal vein and hepatic artery; liver is being dissected, and significant bleeding can occur
Anhepatic phase: From the moment the hepatic venous inflow is being clamped up to graft reperfusion; the IVC is clamped causing a decrease in cardiac output (CO).
Neo-hepatic phase: It begins from the moment of liver reperfusion; resumption of flow in the portal vein and IVC; complicated by post-reperfusion syndrome (PRS) or bleeding from vascular anastomosis (IVC, hepatic artery or portal vein).

490. **(d). About 50% of the cerebral flow is by the internal carotid artery**
Blood flow to the brain is primarily by the paired internal carotid arteries anteriorly and the paired vertebral arteries posteriorly.
About 70% of cerebral blood flow (CBF) is supplied by the internal carotid arteries.
The anterior and posterior circulations anastomose at the base of the brain to form the Circle of Willis.
There are numerous anatomical variations in the Circle of Willis with an incomplete anastomosis in around 50% individuals.

491. **(c). Reflex tachycardia**
Phenylephrine is an alpha1 agonist with very little beta effect.
Its major action is systemic and pulmonary arterial vasoconstriction, increasing SVR and systemic arterial pressure (systolic, diastolic, and mean). Reflex bradycardia can occur. The increase in pulmonary artery pressure is less pronounced than the increase in aortic pressure.

492. **(c). Acinus**
In contrast to a lobule, an *acinus*, the functional unit of the liver, is defined by a portal tract in the middle and centrilobular veins at the periphery.

493. **(b). Diabetus mellitus**
The donors are further differentiated into standard criteria donors (SCD) or extended criteria donors (ECD), depending on whether the age of the donor is 60 years or more, or the age is 50–59, with the presence of at least two of the following: hypertension, death from cerebrovascular accident and terminal creatinine >1.5 mg/dL

494. **(c). Remimazolam has organ independent elimination**
Remimazolam is the latest drug innovation in anesthesia. It has an organ independent metabolism and is rapidly hydrolyzed by tissue esterases.
Fospropofol is a prodrug that is enzymatically converted to propofol in the liver with a delayed onset of action (4–8 min) and extended duration of action (20–30 min).
Dexmedetomidine is an α_2-adrenoreceptor agonist with sedative, anxiolytic, and analgesic effects. Its effects on respiratory system are minimal, and it does not cause clinically significant respiratory depression.
A similar strategy has been applied to modify etomidate and reduce its adrenal suppression effects. Investigators have developed an ultrarapid metabolizing etomidate named methoxycarbonyletomidate (MOC-etomidate), which is broken down via nonspecific esterases. The in vitro half-life of MOC-etomidate is approximately one-tenth that of its parent compound etomidate.

495. **(a). Sirolimus—Calcineurin inhibitor**
Sirolimus: TOR inhibitor (mammalian target of rapamycin inhibitor). Target of rapamycin is aproptein kinase.
Tacrolimus: Calcineurin inhibitor.

496. **(c). Hypothalamus**
Hypothalamus is the primary central structure regulating temperature.

497. **(a). General anesthesia increases the shivering threshold**
Thresholds for vasoconstriction and shivering are 36.5°C and 36.0°C, respectively. General anesthesia lowers this threshold by 2°C–3°C.

498. **(b). Type B blood has Anti-A antibodies in the plasma.**
- The most common blood group is O
- Type O blood is considered universal donor and can be safely given without risk of reaction due to ABO incompatibility, but reactions due to incompatibility other than ABO exists and should therefore be crossmatched.
- Crossmatch involves adding the donor red cells to recipient's plasma and checking for agglutination.

499. (c). Metabolized by conjugation in the liver
   A. Morphine has low lipid solubility
   B. Poorly bound (20-40%) to plasma proteins
   D. Metabolite morphine-6-glucuronide is the more potent μ-receptor agonist and contributes to morphine's analgesic effects.

500. (c). Carbon monoxide poisoning
   The oxy-hemoglobin dissociation curve is shifted to:

Left	Right
Fall in temperature	Rise in temperature
Fall in H⁺ (high pH)	Rise in H⁺ (low pH)
Fall in 2,3- DPG in red blood cells	Rise in 2,3 - DPG in red blood cells
Stored blood	Increasing CO_2 tension
Carbon monoxide poisoning	Pregnancy (normal pregnancy, P50 is higher)
Fetal hemoglobin	Hemoglobin S
Methemoglobinemia	After acclimatisation at high altitudes

501. (b). Closing capacity is increased
   - In elderly, body water is reduced, and affects volume of distribution of certain drugs
   - FRC increases but much lesser than the increase in closing capacity.
   - Creatinine clearance declines with age.

502. (c). ADH secretion is increased
   Stress response leads to an
   - Increased secretion of ACTH, Cortisol, ADH, Renin, Aldosterone, Growth hormone, Prolactin and Glucagon
   - Decreased secretion of Insulin and Testosterone.

503. (c). Oxygen
   Paramagnetism is a property by which certain materials are attracted by an externally applied magnetic field. Materials which display this property are called paramagnetic. Oxygen is attracted to the magnetic field because it has two electrons in unpaired orbits which cause it to possess paramagnetic properties. Most other gases used in anesthesia are repelled by the magnetic field or diamagnetic.

504. (b). Is a Mapleson E with an open ended reservoir bag
   - The T-piece though used chiefly in pediatric can be used in adults with a suitable FGF and reservoir volume. A FGF, 2.5–3 times the minute ventilation and a reservoir bag approximating to the tidal volume are required to achieve this.
   - Jackson Rees added a double ended reservoir bag to the tubing of a Mapleson E. The bag acts as a visual monitor during spontaneous breathing and can be used for controlled ventilation
   - It is not an efficient system. A FGF, 2.5 -3 times the minute volume is required to prevent rebreathing.
   - If the reservoir bag is too small, ambient air will be entrained with resultant dilution of the FGF.

505. (d). Increases the risk of awareness during anesthesia
   - Activation of the O_2 emergency flush can deliver 35-75 litres/min of O_2
   - It is not safe to use the flush during anesthesia, as the high flows can result in barotrauma. Also the risk of awareness is increased due to dilution of the anesthetic gas mixture and delivery of 100% O_2
   - The minute volume divider may not function appropriately due to high flows (35-75L/min)
   - Awareness is a risk due to dilution of the anesthetic gas mixture.

506. (b). The vapourization chamber is pressurized to 1550 mmHg (approx 2 bar)
   Desfurane has a saturated vapor pressure of 664 mmHg at 20°C and a boiling point of 23.5°C. In order to overcome these properties, in the Tec 6 vaporizer, the desflurane is heated to a temperature of 39° C with a pressure of 1550 mmHg (approx. 2 bar).
   The percentage control dial calibration is from 0% to 18%, with 1% graduations from 0-10% and 2% graduations from 10–18%
   The Tec 6 vaporizer design is completelydifferent from the previous Tec series, however it can be mounted onto the selectatec system without the use of any special adaptor.

507. (c). Left ventricular failure
   PCWP remains normal in ARDS, Pulmonary hypertension, pulmonary embolism and tricuspid regurgitation. PCWP is increased in left ventricular failure and severe mitral stenosis.

508. (d). For accurate mechanomyography, a preload of 100–300 g must be applied
   A). A nerve stimulator should produce a constant current output over a range of electrical impedance of tissues to which they are applied
   B). A double burst stimulation consists of two 0.2 ms stimuli separated by 750 ms interval
   C). A double burst stimulation is more accurate and also easy to detect visually than a TOF.

509. (d). Recommend a minimum fast of 4 hours for breast milk
   A) It takes about 2 hours for clear fluids to empty from the stomach
   B). For solid food, the guidelines recommend 6–8 hours only if the meal includes fried or fatty food
   C). Milk thickens when mixed with gastric juice and should be regarded as a solid.

510. **(d). The Lack circuit is more efficient for spontaneous ventilation than controlled ventilation**
    A). Mapleson A and D (Lack and Bain) circuits are used co-axially, not B
    B). Mapleson D circuits are actually more efficient when used for controlled ventilation (require < 1 x minute volume) rather than spontaneous.
    C). The Ayres T piece requires 2-3 x minute volume.

511. **(b). Inheritance is by an autosomal dominant mechanism**
    - Malignant hyperthermia is inherited as an autosomal dominant with links to gene loci on chromosomes 17 and 19.
    - Triggering agents include suxamethonium, (which can produce a very rapid onset) halothane, enflurane, isoflurane, desflurane, sevoflurane, methoxyflurane, ether and cyclopropane.
    - The incidence is approximately 1/15,000 anesthetics.
    - Mannitol is present in bottles of Dantrolene to make the solution isotonic.
    - Dantrolene will produce mild muscle weakness even at high doses.

512. **(b). Increase in minute ventilation is caused by increase in tidal volume**
    A). There is an increase in stroke volume more than heart rate.
    B). This is true, thought to be due to a central effect of progesterone
    C). Gastric acidity does not increase.
    D). Gastroesophageal reflux occurs in pregnancy in 80% women, due to the effects of progesterone on the lower oesophageal sphincter and uterus pushing the stomach into a horizontal position but, Gastric emptying is delayed in labor.

513. **(b). The catheter should not be withdrawn through the Touhy needle once it has been threaded beyond the bevel**
    A). To reduce chances of vascular or dural puncture, unilateral block (since catheter can pass through the intervertebral foramen) and knotting, only 3–5 cm of the epidural catheter is left in the epidural space
    B). Withdrawal of the epidural catheter through the Touhy needle after being threaded beyond the bevel can lead to transection or breakage of the catheter. If the need arises to withdraw the catheter, the Touhy needle along with the catheter should be withdrawn together and the epidural catheterization reattempted.
    C). Catheters with a single port at the tip increase incidence of vascular or dural puncture. Because of the 'sharp' point at the end of the catheter. Catheters with side ports have closed rounded end, which reduces the incidence of vascular or dural puncture.
    D). Some catheters are designed to be radio-opaque. They are more rigid then the standard catheters. They are mainly used in patients.

514. **(b). Is lipid soluble**
    A). Fentanyl is a synthetic opioid, with an analgesic potency 100 times that of morphine
    B). It is highly lipid soluble and has a large volume of distribution
    C). After repeated doses or infusion, cumulation does occurs. After a single dose its duration of action is 20-30 minutes due to redistribution
    D). Undergoes hepatic metabolism (N-dealkylation) and is converted to the inactive metabolite, norfentanyl.

515. **(a). Approximately 15% of the resting cardiac output**
    - Cerebral blood flow is autoregulated between a Mean arterial pressure range of 60-160 mmHg, and is very effective in preventing any changes in flow within this range
    - The autonomic nervous system plays a very insignificant role in regulating the cerebral blood flow
    - Regional blood flow increases during increased mental activity, but the total cerebral blood flow remains constant.

516. **(d). It is proportional to the number of dural punctures**
    A). Both Yale & Quincke needles have a higher incidence of PDPH. Because of the bevel which cuts the dural fibers which allows CSF leak
    B). The incidence of PDPH is directly proportional to the size of the needle. A 20G spinal needle causes a 30% incidence, while a 26 G needle has a 1% incidence
    C). The incidence of PDPH is higher in young as compared to elderly population
    D). The incidence of PDPH is increased with multiple dural punctures.

517. **(a). Increased by an increase in carbon dioxide concentration in the arterial blood**
    A). CO_2 reactivity or an increase in cerebral blood flow with changes in $PaCO_2$ occurs between an arterial CO_2 concentration of 40 mmHg to 80 mmHg
    B). The cerebral blood flow is very well autoregulated between a Mean arterial pressure (MAP) of 60–160 mmHg. Any change in systemic BP within this range does not affect the cerebral bood flow
    C). The autonomic nervous system does not play an important role in the regulation of cerebral blood flow
    D). Regional blood flow in the brain is increased during intense mental activity, but total cerebral blood flow remains unchanged.

518. **(d). Inversely proportional to the viscosity**
    Factors that affect laminar flow through a tube are well explained by the Hagen-Poiseuille equation

$$\frac{\Delta P \pi R^4}{8\eta l}$$

The flow is directly proportional to the pressure drop across the tube and the fourth power of the radius. Inversely proportional to the length of the tube and the viscosity of the fluid.

Density does not affect laminar flow. It affects turbulent flow.

519. (a). Makes up 80% hemoglobin at birth
A) HbF forms 80% of hemoglobin at birth
B) It is made of two alpha and two gamma chains
C) By 6 months of age, adult hemoglobin (HbA) completely replaces HbF
D) HbF has a greater affinity for Oxygen than HbA, because it binds stongly with the 2,3-DPG and the oxyhemoglobin dissociation curve is shifted to the left.

520. (d). Forms a cloudy precipitate with thiopentone
In a case of suspected dural puncture, CSF can be identified by:
- CSF feels warm, when it falls onto the skin
- Forms a cloudy precipitate with 2.5% thiopentone
- CSF has sugar, which will show up on a test strip
- CSF is clear, colourless with a pH of 7.33 and does not turn litmus paper pink.

521. (c). Stimulated by decrease in pH
A) Carotid body contains chemoreceptors. It the carotid sinus which contains stretch receptors
B) It's blood supply is approximately 40 times that of the brain at 2000 mL/100 g/min.
C) The carotid body receptors are stimulated by, an increase in $PaCO_2$, a decrease in PaO_2, a decrease in pH, Venous stasis and in cyanide poisoning (where tissue utilization of Oxygen is prevented)
D) Due to the very high blood flow, oxygen needs of the cells are met by dissolved oxygen itself. In cases of carbon monoxide poisoning and anemia, where the dissolved oxygen levels in the blood remain normal, these receptors are not stimulated.

522. (d). There is an increase in intracranial pressure
Valsalva Manoeuvre involves a forced expiration against a closed glottis.
At the onset of straining, the blood pressure rises due to an increase in the intrathoracic pressure which adds to the pressure of blood in the aorta.
Intracranial pressure increases.
The blood pressure then drops due to the decrease in venous return and a subsequent fall in cardiac output due to the raised intrathoracic pressure.
The fall in blood pressure and pulse pressure inhibits the baroreceptors which leads to an increase in peripheral resistance and tachycardia.
At the end of the manoeuvre, the intrathoracic pressure returns to normal, cardiac output is restored, but peripheral vasoconstriction persists. The blood pressure therefore rises above normal and stimulates the baroreceptors which results in bradycardia along with a drop in the blood pressure towards normal.
20-40% of long standing diabetic patients have autonomic neuropathy. In patients with autonomic neuropathy due to any cause, the heart rate changes are absent.

523. (d). The ciliary ganglion
The stellate and celiac ganglia are sympathetic ganglia. The Gasserian ganglion is the fifth cranial nerve ganglion.

524. (d). Prolonged QT is associated with recurrent syncope or sudden death due to ventricular arrhythmias including Torsade de pointes
The Q-T interval on ECG represents the duration of the ventricular systole. It is measured from the beginning of the Q wave to the end of the T wave. Shortened in hypercalcemia, hyperkalemia and digoxin therapy Prolonged in hypocalcemia and hypothermia.
Prolonged Q-T syndromes (Romano Ward syndrome, Jervell Lange Nielson syndrome) are associated with recurrent syncope or sudden death due to ventricular arrhythmias including Ventricular tachycardia and Torsade de pointes.

525. (d). Though widely performed, may be inaccurate in predicting risk from ischemic damage
Allen's test was described originally for assessing arterial flow to the hand in thromboangiitis obliterans.
Modified for assessing the ulnar arterial flow prior to cannulation of the radial artery.
The ulnar and radial arteries are compressed at the wrist and the patient is asked to clench the fist tightly and open the hand, causing blanching. Pressure over the ulnar artery is released. The color of the palm normally takes less than 5-10 seconds to return to normal. If time taken is over 20seconds, it is considered abnormal.
Though widely performed, it is inaccurate in predicting risk from ischemic damage.

526. (b). Argon can accumulate when oxygen concentrators are used with a circle system
An oxygen concentrator is a device that extracts oxygen from atmospheric air. Air is passed under pressure through columns of zeolite which act as a molecular sieve, trapping nitrogen and water vapour while allowing oxygen and trace gases to pass through. The nitrogen is removed by depressurising the column. Two columns are used alternatively, adsorbing and eliminating nitrogen.

The maximum oxygen concentration that is achieved is 95%. The rest includes trace gases, mainly argon. When using low flows in a circle system, the argon gas can cumulate. Higher fresh gas flows are required to avoid this.

Oxygen concentrators range in size from small units for home use to large ones which can supply oxygen to an entire hospital.

527. (b). The ventral primary rami of cervical nerves 5 to 8 (C5-C8), including a greater part of the first thoracic nerve (T1)

The brachial plexus is formed due to fusion of the ventral primary rami of cervical nerves 5 to 8 (C5-C8), including a greater part of the first thoracic nerve (T1). Variable contributions may be from the fourth cervical-C4 (prefixed) and the second thoracic -T2 (postfixed) nerves.

528. (b). The anterior division of the inferior trunk

Cervical and thoracic roots form 3 trunks superior, inferior and middle. Each trunk divides as anterior and posterior divisions. The anterior divisions of the superior and middle trunks form the lateral cord of the plexus, the posterior divisions of all 3 trunks form the posterior cord; and the anterior division of the inferior trunk forms the medial cord. The three cords then divide and give rise to the terminal braches of the plexus.

529. (c). At the lateral border of the first rib, behind the clavicle

The roots of the brachial plexus unite to form trunks in the interscalene groove. The trunks (anterior, middle and posterior) divide into anterior and posterior divisions at the lateral border of the first rib, behind the clavicle. These divisions continue into the axilla to form cords, which are named according to their position with respect to axillary artery. Each cord divides into terminal branches near the lower border of the pectoralis muscle.

530. (a). In the supraclavicular approach, the trunks and divisions of the plexus is blocked providing the most widespread surgical anesthesia for the whole arm

Numerous approaches have been described for blocking the brachial plexus. One needs to select the approach based on surgical need and expertise. The roots of the plexus are blocked at the interscalene groove (interscalene approach) in shoulder or proximal humerus surgeries. The supraclavicular approach blocks the trunks and division at the level of the first rib and provides anesthesia for the whole arm. This approach poses a risk of pneumothorax. The infraclavicular approach blocks the cords and is preferred for surgeries of hand and arm, the musculocutaneous nerve is also blocked by this approach. The axillary blocks the terminal branches, the musculocutaneous branch may be spared and may need additional injection in the coracobrachialis muscle.

531. (d). Suprascapular nerve
- The nerves that arise from the roots of the brachial plexus includes long thoracic nerve, dorsal scapular nerve and nerve to subclavius.
- The suprascapular nerve is a branch of the upper trunk of brachial plexus and supplies the supra and infraspinatus muscles.
- The Medial and lateral pectoral nerve arise from the respective cords.

532. (d). Elderly

Globe injury occurs in 1,000 to 1:12,000 cases. Though it was believed that the incidence of globe injury is higher in myopes because of a bigger globe, it is seen that myopia is only a significant risk factor for inadvertent perforation when associated with staphyloma. Enophthalmos and prior scleral buckle procedure is also associated with increased risk of perforation.

533. (c). Conjunctival chemosis is less than peribulbar block

Retrobulbar block is produced by injecting the local anesthetic into the space behind the eye within the muscle cone. This clock has advantage of rapid onset of block with small volume of drug. The irsk of the block includes hematoma, scleral perforation and bradycardia due to oculocardiac reflex. However, the risk of chemosis is higher in peribulbar block (17.4%) when compared to retrobulbar blocks (7.1%).

534. (d). It is also effective in strabismus surgeries

Sub-Tenons block is also known as episcleral block. It is most widely used regional anesthesia for cataract surgeries in the United Kingdom. The space between the Tenons capsule and the globe is known as episcleral space. After anesthetizing the conjunctiva with topical anesthesia, a conjunctival incision is made in the infero nasal quadrant. With the help of a blunt tip cannula, local anesthetic is deposited in the sub-Tenon's space. The local anesthetic deposited in this space produces akinesia and anesthesia by diffusing into intra and extra conal zones. This technique is not usually associated with complication see with needle-based blocks like perforation of eyeball and optic nerve damage. Chemosis, sub conjunctival hemorrhage are common complications associated with the block. This block is effective in varied eye surgeries like vitreoretinal surgery, strabismus correction, and trabeculectomy.

535. **(b). Excessive sound energy can cause mechanical and thermal damage to the eye**
    The orbit is well suited for USG examination and is routinely done in ophthalmic practice. The eye is a delicate organ and excessive sound energy can cause thermal; and mechanical damage. Ophthalmic rated transducers limit transducer power output when used for eye examination mode. USG guided block helps in real time visualization of the needle trajectory and thus limit complications. Following local anesthetic injection during peri/retro bulbar blocks an echo void 'T' sign is seen is seen outlining the optic nerve which correlates well with block success.

536. **(b). Procaine**
    German Surgeon August Bier first described the Biers block in 1908 using procaine. Due to adverse effect of procaine, the local failed to gain popularity. Homes reintroduced the technique in 1963 using lignocaine instead of procaine.

537. **(d). Anemia**
    Vascular reasons like peripheral vascular disease, Raynaud's phenomenon, Systemic illness like Scleroderma, Hypertension >200 mm Hg, morbid obesity, Local reasons like lymphedema, infection in the limb, Hematological reasons (Sickle cell disease or trait, methaemoglobinaemia), Pagets diease, Allergy to local anaesthetic, Children (relative contraindication), Procedures needed in both arms, Uncooperative or confused patient.

538. **(b). 7.8**
    - The concentration pf local anesthetic base in solution is equal to the concentration of charged ion at certain hydrogen ion concentration The logarithm of this hydrogen ion concentration is Pk_a.
    - The Pk_a of lidocaine is 7.8 and that of bupivacaine is 8.1.

539. **(c). Bupivacaine**
    - Local anesthetic are classified as low intermediate and high potency based on their relative conduction blocking potency of C fibers in vitro.
    - Procaine has low potency. Mepivacaine, Prilocaine, Chloroprocaine, Lidocaine have intermediate potency. While Tetracaine, Bupivacaine, and Etidocaine have high potency.

540. **(c). Brachial plexus block**
    The duration of action following bupivacaine administration for brachial plexus block averages around 10 hours. The prolonged block noted following brachial plexus could be related to the slow rate of vascular absorption, larger doses of drug required for the block and long segment of nerve exposed to the local anesthetic.

541. **(d). 35 to 55 mg/kg of lidocaine with adrenaline**
    Tumescent anesthesia is a form of local anesthesia for performing liposuction and other soft tissue surgeries with minimal anesthesia and blood loss. Doses of 35 to 55 mg/kg of lidocaine with adrenaline have been safely injected in the subcutaneous tissues. Infiltration of such large volume makes the tissue swell or tumescent. The added epinephrine causes vasoconstriction and reduces the absorption of lidocaine. Removal of subcutaneous fat during surgery further limits the systemic absorption of the local anesthetic. However monitoring for systemic signs of local anesthetic toxicity is essential.

542. **(a). Intercostal nerve blockade**
    The systemic absorption of local anesthetic is determined by the site of injection, addition of vasoconstrictor and dosage and volume of local anesthetic used.
    The absorption of local anesthetic is highest after intercostal nerve blockade, followed in the order of decreasing concentration by injection into caudal epidural space, lumbar epidural space, brachial plexus and subcutaneous tissue.

543. **(c). It is not recommended that bupivacaine induced ventricular arrhythmia be treated with lidocaine or amiodarone**
    - Methemoglobinemia is a unique side effect associated with administration of large dose of prilocaine. O toluidine, a metabolite of prilocaine oxidizes hemoglobin to methemoglobin. Methylene blue administration intravenously helps in treating sever methemoglobinemia.
    - The two active metabolites of lidocaine are monoethylglycylxylidide (MEGX) and glycylxylidide (GX). The potential for toxicity with lidocaine infusions is increased in neonates due to accumulation of its principal metabolite monoethylglycylxylidide (MEGX), which can cause seizures.
    - Cardiovascular collapse seen with bupivacaine overdose is treated with resuscitation drugs like epinephrine, atropine, vasopressin and intralipid formulations. It is not recommended that bupivacaine induced ventricular arrhythmia be treated with lidocaine or amiodarone.

544. **(d). Loss of CSF flow leads to compensatory venous vasoconstriction which adds to symptoms of PDPH**
    Cerebrospinal fluid (CSF) leaks from the dural puncture causing a decrease in CSF volume and pressure. This leads to compensatory dilatation of the cerebral ves-

sels, which contributes to PDPH. The CSF volume loss also causes a downward pull on pain of the brain and pain sensitive structures. Change in concentration of substance P and the regulation of neurokinin 1 receptors is also responsible for PDPH.

545. **(b). Quincke**
    - Atraumatic spinal needles cause separation of dural fibers resulting in early healing. E.g., Sprotte, Cappe, Deutsch, Whitacre and Atraucan needles.
    - Traumatic needle on the other hand cut the dural fibers leading to a larger defect, e.g., Ferguson, Lutz, Brace, Quincke, Greene, Hingson and Rovenstine.

546. **(c). In Ninety percent of the cases the headache starts within 72 hours of the dural puncture**
    - Though the incidence of unintentional dural puncture during labor analgesia is 0.15–1.5%, the incidence of PDPH is 50–80% in these women.
    - In 66% of cases, the symptoms start within 48 hours, while in 90% of patients are symptomatic with 72 hours of dural puncture.
    - Current evidence does not support the prophylactic use of any measure including epidural blood patch.
    - Epidural blood patch is the gold standard for treatment of PDPH with completer relief in 32 and partial relief in 73.

547. **(a). Spinal nerve that exit the cord are numbered as thoracic, lumbar, sacral based on the vertebra above**
    - As the vertebral column grows, the spinal cord is left behind as a result it tends to 'ascend'. In adults the spinal cord ends at the lower border of of L1 and the Dural sac ends at lower border of S2.
    - The spinal nerves exit at each level. The 1–7 cranial nerves are numbered as per vertebra below. The C8 leaves between C7 and T1. All thoracic, lumbar and sacral nerves are according to the vertebra above.

548. **(b). Supraorbital, supratrochlear, auriculotemporal, zygomaticotemporal, greater and lesser occipital nerves**
    Complete scalp block includes blocking six nerves: supraorbital, supratrochlear, auriculotemporal, zygomaticotemporal, greater and lesser occipital nerves.

549. **(b). Greater occipital**
    The branches from the superficial cervical plexus include lesser occipital (C2, C3), great auricular (C2, C3), transverse cervical (C2, C3), and supraclavicular nerves (C3, C4). Greater occipital does not arise from the cervical plexus. It is spinal nerve, the medial branch of the dorsal primary ramus of cervical spinal nerve 2.

550. **(d). Lateral femoral cutaneous nerve**
    "Meralgia paresthetica" is a condition in which there exist compression of the lateral femoral cutaneous nerve leading to sensory disturbance. The nerve is a purely sensory nerve that arises from L2-3 roots of the lumbar plexus. It provides sensation to anterolateral thigh.

551. **(c). Pudendal nerve**
    - The sacral plexus is formed by L5-S4 roots.
    - The nerves that arise from the sacral plexus include the superior gluteal nerve (L4-S1), inferior gluteal nerve (L5-S2), sciatic nerve, posterior femoral nerve (S1-3), and pudendal nerve (S1-S4).
    - Genitofemoral nerve, Saphenous nerve, Ilioinguinal nerve arise from the Lumbar plexus.

552. **(c). Acoustic shadows of the transverse process**
    During longitudinal ultrasound image of the spine, the acoustic shadow of the transversus processes produces the trident sign.

553. **(d). During femoral block, depositing the local anesthetic only anteriorly to the nerve results in fewer needle redirection and greater satisfaction then depositing the drug circumferentially of the nerve**
    The femoral nerve is a superficial block performed using a high frequency linear probe. The nerve appears as a triangular **hyperechoic** structure in the **transverse** section, and is blocked using an in plane technique. The nerve lies lateral to the artery and **deep to the fascia lata and iliaca** and on the anterior aspect of the iliopsoas muscle. A previous study has shown that depositing the local anesthetic only anteriorly to the nerve results in fewer needle redirection and greater satisfaction then depositing the drug circumferentially of the nerve.

554. **(b). Fascia iliaca compartment block**
    The fascia iliaca compartment block (FICB) is a potential space between the fascial iliaca anteriorly and iliacus and psoas muscle posteriorly. The FICB blocks the femoral nerve, the lateral cutaneous nerve of thigh and the obturator nerve.

555. **(c). Preventive epidural analgesia using Ketamine and Local anesthetic**
    - As per the clinical narrative review published in 2018, the institution of preoperative epidural catheter prior to amputation and its continuation in the immediate postoperative period reduced perioperative opioid consumption (Level II).
    - Optimized preoperative epidural or intravenous patient-controlled analgesia starting 48 hours and continuing for 48 hours postoperatively decreased PLP at 6 months (Level II).

- Preventive role of epidural LA with ketamine (Level II) reduced persistent pain at 1 year and LA with calcitonin decreased PLP at 12 months (Level II).
- Peripheral nerve catheters have opioid sparing effect in the immediate postoperative period in postamputation patients (Level I), but evidence is low for the prevention of PLP (Level III).
- Gabapentin did not reduce the incidence or intensity of postamputation pain (Level II).

556. (a). Diagnosis is dependent on triad of back pain, fever, and paralysis

The classical triad of symptoms includes: back pain, fever and neurological deterioration, but is present only in 10-15% of patients at first contact

As severe back pain is the most common symptom, every patient with back pain, fever and predisposing risk factors should be evaluated as suspected of SEA.

Four stages may be identified in SEA development: 1) back pain at the level of the affected spine, fever, spine tenderness; 2) radicular pain 3) neurological deficits such as hypoaesthesia, motor weakness, bowel or bladder dysfunction; 4) paralysis. The rate of progression from one stage to another and the duration of symptoms vary from a few hours to several days. The diagnosis is based on neuroimaging and early suspicion.

Staphylococcus aureus is responsible for about 70% of SEA cases.

557. (d). Descending portion of the pelvic colon
- This block targets the liver, gallbladder, omentum, pancreas, mesentery, and the digestive tract from the stomach all the way to the transverse large colon.
- The indications for a celiac plexus block include treatment of intractable intra-abdominal pain, including pain in the setting of malignant and benign neoplasms involving the pancreas, biliary tree, retroperitoneal organs, and other abdominal organs.

558. (a). C5-T1 anterior primary

The brachial plexus is formed by the anterior primary rami of C5 through T1 and provides sensory and motor innervation of the upper extremity. The brachial plexus is divided, proximally to distally into rami/roots, trunks, divisions, cords, and terminal branches.

559. (c). Check his renal function
- Gabapentin doses needs adjustment depending on creatinine clearance.
- Gabapentin or pregabalin may be better tolerated in cirrhosis because of non-hepatic metabolism and a lack of anti-cholinergic side effects.
- Gabapentin can interact with losartan, ethacrynic acid, caffeine, phenytoin, mefloquine, magnesium oxide, cimetidine, naproxen, sevelamer and morphine. Gabapentin use is contraindicated in patients with myasthenia gravis or myoclonus.

560. (a). Characterized by disabling pain, swelling, vasomotor instability, sudomotor abnormality, and impairment of motor function
- Complex regional pain syndrome (CRPS) is a neuropathic pain disorder defined by the presence of distinct clinical features, including allodynia, hyperalgesia, sudomotor and vasomotor abnormalities, and trophic changes. The pain experienced is disproportionate to the degree of tissue injury and persists beyond the normal expected time for tissue healing.
- There are two subtypes: type I, formerly known as reflex sympathetic dystrophy, and type II, formerly known as causalgia. Type I occurs in the absence of nerve trauma, while type II occurs in the setting of known nerve trauma.
- CRPS is further subdivided into "warm" versus "cold" and sympathetically-maintained versus sympathetically-independent, which may affect prognosis and treatment options.
- The most optimal management would include an interprofessional approach including physical and occupational therapy, pharmacotherapy, behavioral therapy, and interventions.

561. (d). Bony metastasis

Sympathetic blocks like lumbar sympathetic blocks is the treatment modality for Raynaud's.
- The most common complication of herpes zoster in immunocompetent patients is postherpetic neuralgia (PHN). Sympathetic blocks have been traditionally used for patients with herpes zoster and PHN with three different therapeutic goals: pain relief during acute herpes zoster, pain relief during PHN, and prevention of PHN by treating patients with acute zoster.
- Sphenopalatine Ganglion block for the treatment of acute migraine headache
- Bony metastasis pain: Treatment options are: use of non-steroidal anti-inflammatory drugs (NSAIDs), opioids, bisphosphonates, tricyclic antidepressants, corticosteroids, growth factors and signaling molecules, ET-1 receptor antagonists, radiotherapy as well as surgical management.

562. (d). Constipation

Fibromyalgia is a syndrome characterized by chronic widespread pain at multiple tender points, joint stiffness, and systemic symptoms (e.g., mood disorders, fatigue, cognitive dysfunction, and insomnia) without a well-defined underlying organic disease.

563. **(a). Educating the patient regarding the condition plays an important role**
   - It is important that patients with fibromyalgia understand their illness before the prescription of any medications.
   - The medications that have been well studied and consistently effective are certain antidepressants and anticonvulsants. The antidepressants include tricyclic medications, like amitriptyline and other selective serotonin reuptake inhibitors (SSRIs) and norepinephrine reuptake inhibitors (SNRIs) including duloxetine and milnacipran.

564. **(a). Ulnar**
   The interscalene block covers most of the brachial plexus, sparing the ulnar (C8-T1) nerve. It is a great block for distal clavicle, shoulder, and proximal humerus procedures.

565. **(c). T9-L2**
   The artery of Adamkiewicz typically arises from the left side of the aorta between T8 and L2 (usually T9 to T12, although the artery of Adamkiewicz is found above T8 in about 15% of people), and has been documented as having a diameter anywhere from 0.6 to 1.8 mm.
   Clinical implications:
   Anterior cord syndrome (also called anterior spinal artery syndrome) most commonly occurs due to an interrupted supply of the anterior spinal artery or the Artery of Adamkiewicz (its major supplier), which has a less efficient supply compared to the 2 posterolateral spinal arteries. This commonly is caused by atherosclerotic disease, trauma (surgical instrumentation or direct injury by a disc or bone fragment), hypotension (for example, from blood loss in open surgery like bowel resection).
   Transforaminal epidural steroid injections are commonly used to treat radicular pain, and there have been case reports of spinal cord infarction and acute paraplegia following this procedure.

566. **(b). Lateral**
   Coeliac plexus approaches are anterior and posterior. Posterior approach is divided into retrocrural or transcrural (also known as anterocrural).

567. **(a). Consists of three major measures to be assessed**
   - The McGill Pain Questionnaire, also known as McGill Pain Index, is a scale of rating pain developed at McGill University by Melzack and Torgerson in 1971.
   - Among the words, sections of these words signify different components of pain, namely, Sensory (sections 1-10), Affective (sections 11-15), Evaluative (section 16), and Miscellaneous (sections 17-20).Thus it's a multidimensional pain scale. It is a widely used scale.

568. **(a). Pain caused by stimuli that are usually not painful**
   Allodynia is a pain due to a stimulus which does not normally provoke pain and can be either thermal or mechanical.

569. **(b). Is usually self-limiting**

570. **(d). Capable of encoding stimulus intensity within the noxious range**
   - Noxious stimuli are transduced into electrical signals in free "unencapsulated" nerve endings that have branched from the main axon and terminate in the wall of arterioles and surrounding connective tissue, and may innervate distinct regions in the dermis and epidermis
   - Nociceptors are divided into A delta, A beta and C fibers.
   - C fiber is the only unmyelinated nociceptor. It is high threshold receptor
   - A delta is both high and low threshold receptor, while A beta is a low threshold receptor.
   - Nociceptors are sensitive to noxious stimulus or to a stimulus that would become noxious if prolonged, capable of encoding stimulus intensities if within noxious range.

571. **(c). Opioid induced hypoalgesia**
   - *Tolerance* is defined as a decreased subjective and objective effect of the same amount of opioids used over time, which concomitantly requires an increasing amount of the drug to achieve the same effect. Although tolerance to most of the side effects of opioids (e.g., respiratory depression, sedation, nausea) does appear to occur routinely, there is less evidence for clinically significant tolerance to opioids- analgesic effects
   - *Physical dependence* represents a characteristic set of signs and symptoms (opioid withdrawal) that occur with the abrupt cessation of an opioid (or rapid dose reduction and/or administration of an opioid antagonist).
   - Pain and addiction are not mutually exclusive and some patients who are treated for pain do develop severe behavioral disturbances indicative of a comorbid addictive disorder.

572. **(d). IV Morphine/ IV Fentanyl in aliquots titrating the analgesic to keep the respiratory rate between 20 to 25**
   The character of postoperative pain may shift for instance from predominantly neuropathic to post-surgical nociceptive pain. The possibility of intraoperative withdrawal should be kept in mind. It typically presents as hemodynamic instability accompanied

by autonomic hyperactivity, reflected as tachycardia and hypo- or hypertension. The pupils are frequently dilated and patients will often have gastric hypersecretion and sweating. One method of dosing the analgesics toward the end of the procedure includes reversing neuromuscular blocking agents and then titrating the analgesia to respiratory rate.

573. **(c). Proceed with surgery. Patient should be counselled and observed**

Horner's syndrome results from paralysis of the ipsilateral sympathetic cervical chain (stellate ganglion) caused by surgery, drugs (mainly high concentrations of local anesthetics), local compression (hematoma or tumor), or inadequate perioperative positioning of the patient. It occurs in 100% of the patients with an interscalene block of the brachial plexus and can also occur in patients with other types of supraclavicular blocks.

574. **(b). Can be because of triple crush mechanism**
- Persistent phrenic nerve palsy after interscalene block is a complication that has recently gained wider recognition, and its incidence has been estimated from case series data to range from 1 in 2,000 up to 1 in 100.
- Causes are direct needle trauma, Intraneural injection, LA myotoxicity, "Double crush" syndrome—due to previous cervical spine stenosis along with nerve trauma, "Triple crush" mechanism that includes pressure ischemia resulting from high volumes of local anesthetic injected within the tight confines of the interscalene sheath.
- Causes of persistent phrenic nerve palsy differ from those implicated in transient phrenic nerve palsy, and thus it cannot be assumed that strategies to reduce the risk of the latter will also reduce the risk of the former.

575. **(d). Injection of LA agent at superior trunk**

Strategies for reducing phrenic nerve palsy and its clinical impact while ensuring adequate analgesia for shoulder surgery are:
- Targeting suprascapular nerve and axillary nerveas an alternative to brachial plexus block
- Limiting the volume and concentration of local anaesthetic agent
- Injection of LA agent 4 mm lateral to brachial plexus nerve sheaths called as periplexus block or extrafascial block
- Injection of LA agent at superior trunk
- Injection of LA agent away from C5–C6 root, that is at C7 root
- In case of use of catheter, volume of infusion less than 2 mL/hr.

576. **(a). Infraorbital nerve block**
- *Cleft Lip:* As it involves mainly the upper lip, the following nerves carry the pain sensation:
- *The infraorbital nerve:* A branch of the maxillary division of the trigeminal nerve. It supplies not only the upper lip, but much of the skin of the face between the upper lip and the lower eyelid, except for the bridge of the nose.
- *The external nasal nerve*: A branch of the ophthalmic nerve that supplies the integument of the ala and tip of the nose.
- *Cleft Palate:* The pain sensation from the palate is carried by the following nerves (all are branches of the maxillary division of trigeminal nerve):
  - The lesser palatine nerve: Supplies the soft palate, tonsil, and uvula.
  - The greater palatine nerve: A branch of the pterygopalatine ganglion, supplies the gums, the mucous membrane and glands of the hard palate, and communicates in front with the terminal filaments of the nasopalatine nerve.
  - Nasopalatine nerve: Supplies the palatal structures around the upper central and lateral incisors and the canines (the upper front six teeth).

577. **(c). The pain of early labour is referred to T10-T12 dermatomes such that pain is felt in the lower abdomen, sacrum and back**
- Visceral pain
- Visceral pain is transmitted by small unmyelinated 'C' fibers which travel with sympathetic fibers and pass through the uterine, cervical and hypogastric nerve plexuses into the main sympathetic chain. The pain fibers from the sympathetic chain enter the white rami communicantes associated with T10 to L1 spinal nerves and pass via their posterior nerve roots to synapse in the dorsal horn of the spinal cord. Some fibers cross over at the level of the dorsal horn with extensive rostral and caudal extension resulting in poorly localised pain. The pain of early labour is referred to T10-T12 dermatomes such that pain is felt in the lower abdomen, sacrum and back. This pain is dull in character and is not always sensitive to opioid drugs; the response to opioids depends on the route of administration.
- Somatic pain
- Somatic pain is transmitted by fine, myelinated rapidly transmitting 'A delta' fibers. Transmission occurs via the pudendal nerves and perineal branches of the posterior cutaneous nerve of the thigh to S2 - S4 nerve roots. Somatic fibers from the cutaneous branches of the ilioinguinal and genitofemoral nerves also carry afferent fibers to L1 and L2. Somatic pain occurs closer to delivery, is sharp in character and easily localised to the

vagina, rectum and perineum. It radiates to the adjacent dermatomes T10 and L1 and compared to visceral pain, is more resistant to opioid drugs. All resulting nerve impulses (visceral and somatic) pass to dorsal horn cells where they are processed and transmitted to the brain via the spino-thalamic tract. Transmission to the hypothalamic and limbic systems accounts for the emotional and autonomic responses associated with pain.

578. **(b). Patient controlled epidural analgesia with a background infusion of 8 mL/hr of 0.1% bupivacaine + Fentanyl 2 mcg/mL with a top ups of 2 mL of 0.1% bupivacaine**
    - Epidural analgesia is the most effective method of providing pain relief in labour and involves injecting local anaesthetic close to the nerves that transmit pain.
    - Low dose local anaesthetic and opioid mixtures; typically 10–15 mL 0.1% bupivacaine with 2 mcg/mL fentanyl provide excellent analgesia while preserving motor function with the mother more likely to mobilize during labour or deliver without assistance. Continuous epidural infusions are associated with more motor block than either top-ups or PCEA. PCEA in labour is set up with a small background infusion and tops up that are smaller in volume than those usually administered by midwives or anesthetists, but which can be administered more often. It results in satisfactory analgesia with reduced overall dose of bupivacaine and fentanyl. The sympathetic blockade accompanying low-dose epidural top-ups is slow in onset and seldom extensive. Maternal hypotension in these circumstances is usually associated with aorto-caval compression.
    - Continuous spinal analgesia is provided by either intermittent bolus or continuous infusion techniques and may be preferred in cases of accidental dural puncture. It is used when other methods of pain relief are not available or in a mother in the very advanced first stage of labor or for high-risk maternities. CSA with microcatheters offers some advantages over the single shot spinal or the continuous epidural techniques but it is associated with complications such as cauda equina syndrome and may be inherently more dangerous than the other two techniques.

579. **(a). Inferonasal**

580. **(a). Supraclavicular brachial plexus block**
    In Supraclavicular approach, brachial plexus is seen posterolateral to subclavian artery in t(he form of bunches). The pleura and the 1st rib is also well seen.

    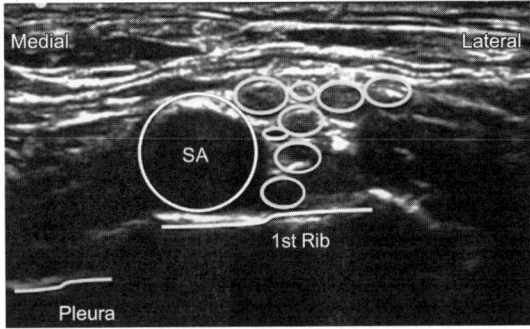

    In Infraclvicular approach, brachial plexus is deeper due to presence of pectorals muscle. The nerves surround the axillary artery.

    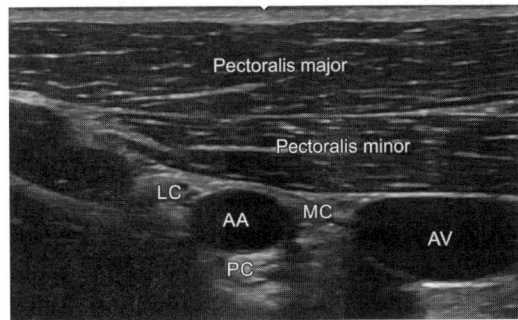

    The pleura is not seen in axillary plexus and interscalene block.

581. **(b). Anterolateral forearm**
    If musculocutaneous is not blocked, sparing of anterolateral forearm will occur.

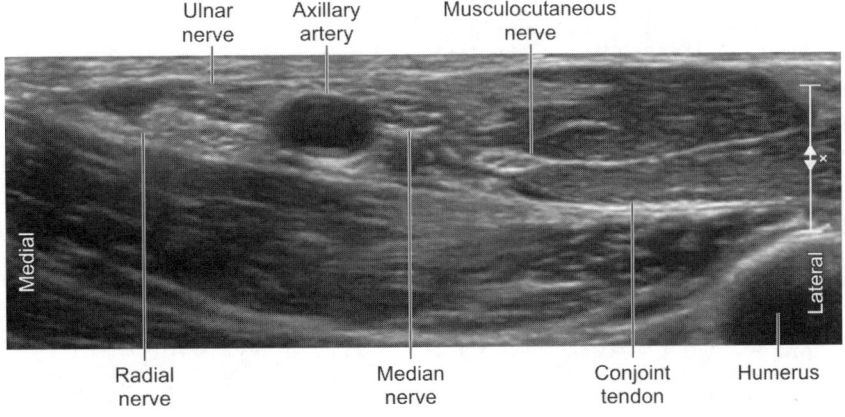

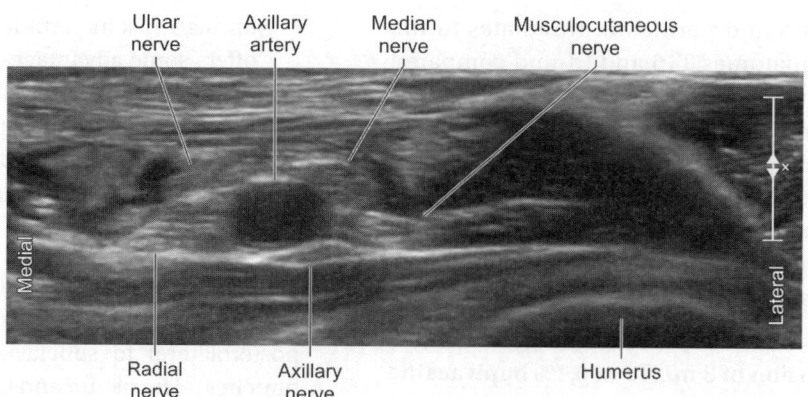

582. (d). Co-loading of fluid during spinal anesthesia along with aliquots of ephedrine or phenylephrine if required
- IV fluid preloading or coloading may be used to reduce the frequency of maternal hypotension after spinal anesthesia for cesarean delivery. **Do not delay the initiation of spinal anesthesia in order to administer a fixed volume of IV fluid.**
- Either IV ephedrine or phenylephrine may be used for treating hypotension during neuraxial anesthesia. In the absence of maternal bradycardia, consider selecting phenylephrine because of improved fetal acid-base status in uncomplicated pregnancies.

583. (a). Pencil point needle
If spinal anesthesia is chosen, use pencil-point spinal needles instead of cutting-bevel spinal needles.

584. (b). PCM + weak opioid
Provision of adequate analgesia is important in the post-operative period as well, since the pain has been shown to increase the risk of premature labour. Regional nerve or plexus blockade or epidural analgesia can provide excellent post-operative analgesia and reduce the risk of opioid-induced hypoventilation when compared with intravenous opioids. Opioids can be used, as needed, to control post-operative pain. Paracetamol is the analgesic of choice for the treatment of mild to moderate pain during any stage of pregnancy.

NSAIDs should be avoided, especially after 32 weeks of gestation, because they may cause premature closure of the fetal ductus arteriosus (if given for more than 48 h). They are also associated with oligohydramnios with reduced foetal renal function.
Only PCM will be inadequately treat severe pain. Additional short term weak opioid will be needed to control severe pain.

585. (a). Subcostal TAP block with catheter with post op IV Patient control Analgesia
Since patient is on warfarin and INR on day of surgery is 1.6, epidural analgesia will be contraindicated in view of risk of epidural hematoma.
Ultrasound guided Truncal blocks are superficial, safe and effective blocks. Truncal block are used as an alternative analgesia technique to epidural in abdominal surgeries.
Since the patient also has a component of COPD, post oertative pain relief and pulmonary rehabilitation is extremely important. Among the truncal blocks bilateral subcoastal TAP block covers the segment from T6 to T9. Hence subcoastal TAP block will be the block of choice over lateral TAP block that covers T10 to L1 and posterior TAP block that covers T 9 to L1 segment. Since the patient is on chronic opioid therapy, patient will need regional analgesia to decrease the need of opioid and its side effects.

586. (a). Upper molars

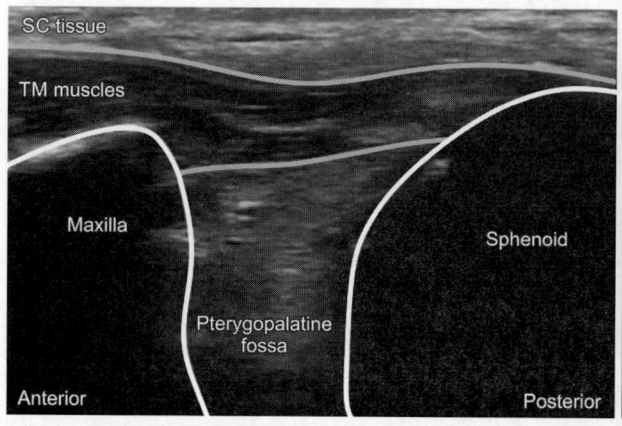
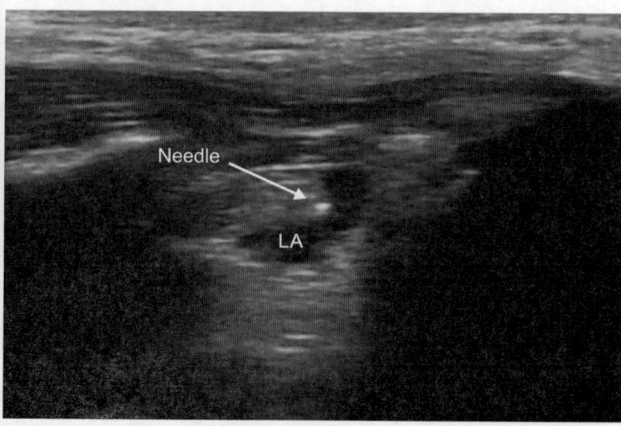

- At the upper part of the pterygopalatine fossa, the maxillary nerve is accessible for a complete maxillary nerve block. The areas supplied by this nerve are lower eyelid, ala of the nose, cheek, upper lip, cutaneous zygomatic, and temporal zone, superior teeth, palatine bone and maxillary bone
- In children, bilateral maxillary nerve blocks improve perioperative analgesia and favor the early resumption of feeding following repair of congenital cleft palate. Many other procedures may benefit from a maxillary nerve block, such as maxillary trauma (LeFort I), maxillary osteotomy, or the diagnostic and therapeutic management of trigeminal neuralgias.

587. (c). Use of low dose opioid

Rapid sequence spinal technique consists of a no-touch spinal technique, consideration of omission of the spinal opioid, limiting spinal attempts, allowing the start of surgery before full establishment of the spinal block, and being prepared for conversion to general anesthesia if there are delays or problems.

588. (a). Sacral cornua

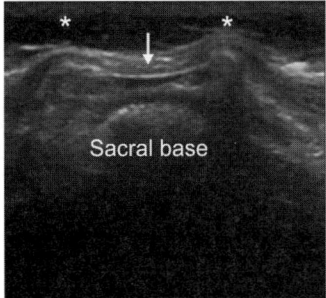 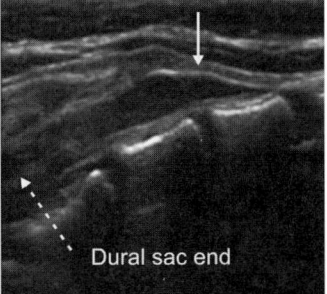

- Ultrasound images during caudal block
- The "frog eye sign" of bilateral sacral cornuae (asterisks) and "hump" of the sacrococcygeal ligament (white arrow) are seen in the transverse plane.
- The anechoic caudal space is seen between the hyperechoic sacro-coccygeal ligament (white arrow) and the dorsum of the pelvic surface of the sacrum in the longitudinal plane.

589. (b). It is an aniline derivative
- Paracetamol is virtually the sole survivor of the so-called "aniline derivatives" or "aniline analgesics" which are acetanilide, phenacetin and paracetamol (acetaminophen).
- Following oral administration it is rapidly absorbed from the gastrointestinal tract, its systemic bioavailability being dose-dependent and ranging from 70 to 90%. Its rate of oral absorption is predominantly dependent on the rate of gastric emptying.
- Paracetamol is extensively metabolized (predominantly in the liver), the major metabolites being the sulphate and glucuronide conjugates. Large doses of paracetamol (overdoses) cause acute hepatic necrosis as a result of depletion of glutathione and of binding of the excess reactive metabolite to vital cell constituents. This damage can be prevented by the early administration of sulfhydryl compounds such as methionine and N-acetylcysteine.

590. (a). Abducens
- Abducens nerve palsy presenting as diplopia is a rare but serious complication of intracranial hypotension from CSF leak. Among the cranial nerves causing ophthalmolplegia, the abducens or the sixth cranial nerve is the most frequently involved with horizontal diplopia and blurred vision. The patients with cranial nerve palsy secondary to intracranial hypotension, 83% of patients had abducens (VI) nerve palsies, 14% had oculomotor (III) nerve palsies, and 7% had trochlear (IV) nerve paresis. Abducens nerve palsy due to intracranial hypotension is a benign condition and about 80% of patients recover spontaneously.
- The abducens nerve is most sensitive to intracranial hypotension. This is not due to its longer course as was earlier believed but due to three acute angulation points between the dural entrance point and its anastomosis with the periarterial sympathetic plexus.

591. (d). May cause withdrawal symptoms in morphine addicts
- Buprenorphine is a thebaine derivative.
- The respiratory depressant action is rare as it has got a ceiling effect but when present is difficult to antagonise with naloxone.
- Oral bioavailability is poor. So, no oral formulations are available. Transdermal patches, sublingual tablets and intravenous/intramuscular formulations are available.
- If buprenorphine is started in opioid-dependent individuals, it will displace the other opioids and cause a phenomenon known as "precipitated withdrawal" which is characterized by a rapid and intense onset of withdrawal symptoms. Individuals must therefore be in a state of mild to moderate withdrawal before starting therapy with buprenorphine.

592. (a). Are reversible in normal kidneys
- All nonsteroidal anti-inflammatory drugs (NSAIDs) inhibit cyclooxygenase, and consequently renal functions dependent upon prostaglandin (PG)

synthesis can be affected. Renal function in normal individuals is relatively independent of the PG system, and thus the NSAIDs don't usually produce any renal dysfunction. However, in some circumstances, inhibition of PG dependent renal functions can produce clinically significant effects. When the kidney is in a salt retaining state or when there is renal vascular damage, NSAIDs can reduce renal blood flow and glomerular filtration rate producing acute renal failure that is reversible upon discontinuation of the drug.

- NSAIDs can also reduce sodium excretion and blunt the diuretic effect of loop diuretics, thus producing or exacerbating edema. They inhibit PG dependent renin secretion occasionally resulting in hyperkalemia, enhance the antidiuretic effects of vasopressin and reduce the antihypertensive efficacy of several drugs.

593. (d). The possibility that the pain is from a pre-existing condition has been excluded

- Persistent postoperative pain has been defined by the International Association for the Study of Pain as a clinical discomfort that lasts more than 2 months postsurgery without other causes of pain such as chronic infection or pain from a chronic condition preceding the surgery.
- According to the International Classification of Diseases, persistent postoperative pain has greater intensity or different pain characteristics than preoperative pain, and is a continuum of acute postoperative pain that may develop after an asymptomatic period.
- International Classification of Diseases defines the duration for persistent postoperative pain at 3 months postsurgery, because healing times differ among different procedures.

594. (b). Gag reflex

- **Gag reflex**—triggered by mechanical and chemical stimulation of areas innervated by the glossopharyngeal nerve, and the efferent motor arc is provided by the vagus nerve and its branches to the pharynx and larynx.
- **Glottic closure reflex**—elicited by selective stimulation of the superior laryngeal nerve, and efferent arc is the recurrent laryngeal nerve. - Exaggeration of this reflex is called laryngospasm.
- **Cough**—the cough receptors located in the larynx and trachea receive afferent and efferent fibers from the vagus nerve.

Glossopharyngeal Nerve can be blocked by one of three.

595. (c). Pasero Opioid-induced Sedation Scale (POSS)

GCS provides a score of the response of the patient to external stimuli.

Level of sedation	Nursing intervention
S-Sleeping, easy to rouse	No action necessary
1-Awake, alert	• No action necessary • May increase sedation
2-Slightly drowsy but easy to rouse	Acceptable, no action necessary
3- Falls asleep during conversation	• Unacceptable • Monitor respiratory status • Notify health care provider to decrease sedation by 25–50%
4-Somnolent, minimal or no response to verbal and physical stimuli	• Stop sedation • Consider using naloxone • Notify health care provider • Monitor respiratory status

596. (c). Adductor canal block

- The rationale behind the adductor canal block (ACB) is that saphenous nerve (sensory nerve) and part of the obturator nerve traveling through the adductor canal of thigh and injecting local anesthetics in the canal will provide adequate analgesia to knee surgeries by blocking these nerves.
- ACB is as effective as Femoral Nerve Block in providing postoperative analgesia after knee surgery. In addition, ACB carries the advantage of preserving or minimally affecting quadriceps strength. Preserving quadriceps strength will facilitate ambulation and postoperative rehabilitation.
- Amount of local anesthetic injection, a recent study by Jœger et al showed that injecting 10 to 30 cc of 0.1% ropivacaine provides adequate pain relief while does not cause motor weakness. However, lower dose of 0.2% ropivaciane has also been used for ACB with satisfactory results.

597. (b). Supraclavicular nerve block

Colloquially known as the "spinal of the arm," the supraclavicular block is advantageous as the brachial plexus nerves are tightly packed in this approach and speed of onset is often rapidly achieved. However, because of this consolidated relationship, consider restricting volumes of local anesthesia to as low as possible to achieve goals, as compression ischemia may occur.

598. (a). Deep peroneal nerve

Achieving a complete ankle block involves anesthesia of all five nerves with the posterior tibial nerve being the major nerve of interest as it innervates all five toes. The cutaneous innervations of these nerves supplying the foot are as follows:

- The posterior tibial nerve provides sensory innervation to the plantar surface of the foot and toes by its three divisions: the medial plantar nerve, lateral plantar nerve, and medial calcaneal nerve.
- The deep peroneal nerve supplies sensation to the dorsum of the foot between the great and second toe.
- The superficial peroneal nerve supplies sensory innervation to the dorsum of the foot and toes, except the web space between the first and second toes and the lateral aspect of the foot.
- The sural nerve provides sensory innervation to the lateral surface of the foot and the heel.
- The saphenous nerve provides sensation to the skin over the medial malleolus, medial surface of the foot up to the medial arch, and to the medial side of the great toe.

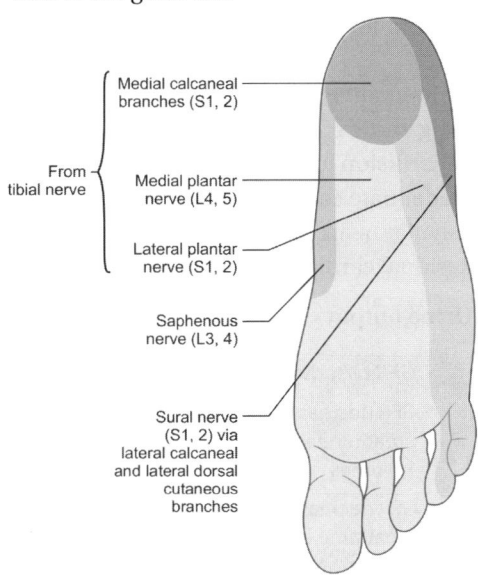

599. (c). Bupivaccaine

Name	Duration	pKa	Partition coefficient	% Protein bound	% Equiv. conc
Lidocaine	1 h	7.8	110	64	1
Prilocaine	1.5 h	7.7	50	55	1
Ropivacaine	2–4 h	8.1	230	94	0.25
Bupivacaine	2–4 h	8.1	560	95	0.25

- Bupivacaine: As the pKa of bupivacaine is 8.1, the onset of action is intermediate or slow. Bupivacaine is the most highly protein-bound (95%) amide local anesthetic, which is the reason for its long duration of action. It is metabolized in the liver by N-dealkylation to pipecolylxy lidine and pipecolic acid.
- Oil-gas p artition coeffcient measures the lipid solubility. It is the main determinant of potency.

600. (a). Lesser than 40%
ppoFEV$_1$ = preopFEV$_1$ × (1 − % of functional lung tissue removed/100)

601. (d). Testing for lung parenchymal function – DLCO
1. RESPIRATORY MECHANICS:
ppoFEV$_1$ = preopFEV$_1$ × (1 − % of functional lung tissue removed/100)
2. CARDIOPULMONARY RESERVE: Calculation of the VO$_2$ max (>15 mL/kg/min) (Staircase climb test > 2 flights, 6 minute walk test, Exercise SpO$_2$ drop <4%)
3. LUNG PARENCHYMAL FUNCTION:
ppo Dlco = preop DLCO × (1 − % of functional lung tissue removed/100)

602. (d). Increase in PCWP, LV, RV, and RA pressures
In classical cardiac tamponade there is an increase in the PCWP, RA, LV and RV pressures to equalise with the pressure in the pericardium. The atrial and ventricular diastolic transmural pressure is zero.

603. (c). Type II
Protamine reactions can range from moderate hypotension to significant hemodynamic alterations. These reactions are categorized into Type I, II, and III.
Type I involves isolated hypotension with normal to low filling pressures.
Type II includes moderate to severe hypotension with features of anaphylactoid reaction like bronchoconstriction.
Type III is caused by heparin-protamine complexes lodged in the pulmonary circulation resulting in raised PA pressures and eventual right heart failure.

604. (c). Higher doses of epinephrine cause reflex bradycardia due to increase in blood pressure
Epinephrine activates α and β receptors. High doses of Epinephrine (>10 ug/min) cause α receptor activation and consequent generalized vasoconstriction. Epinephrine is a potent renal vasoconstrictor. High doses therefore, cause reflex bradycardia as a consequence of the increased blood pressure. Doses between 2-10 ug/minute increase heart rate, contractility and decrease the refractory period of myocardial tissue.

605. (b). The binding of the agonist to the receptor does not cause opening of the channel
Desensitization block occurs when the binding of the receptor to the agonist does not cause the channel to open. Drugs causing densenstization block are volatile anaesthetics, polymyxin B, ethanol, thiopental and local anaesthetics.

606. (c). Important causes are dapsone and benzocaine in susceptible patients
- Methemoglobinemia results from the oxidization of the usual ferrous (Fe^{2+}) atom to the ferric (Fe^{3+})

form and is unable to bind to oxygen with the same affinity resulting in decreased oxygen delivery in the body.
- Patient may appear blue due to the blue brown color of Methemoglobin.
- This cyanosis is not reversed by supplemental oxygen and the treatment involves converting Methemoglobin to Hb using methylene blue.

607. (a). 21.5 and 23.3 mmol/Lit of blood respectively

608. (c). 12–15%

609. (d). Nitrous oxide
- All anesthetic agents in general suppress the cerebral metabolic rate (CMR) mainly by acting on the electrophysiologic function.
- Exceptions to this are ketamine and nitrous oxide.
- Barbiturates, propofol, etomidate, most inhalational agents suppress EEG activity and hence suppress CMR.
- Any increase in the concentration of these drugs beyond the plasma concentration required for suppression of the EEG will not cause a further decrease in CMR.

610. (a). $V_E = V_A + fx\ V_D$
The portion of the tidal volume that reaches the alveoli is termed as alveolar ventilation. Its relation with minute ventilation is best described as
$V_E = V_A + fx\ V_D$
The normal alveolar ventilation is 5 L/min which is almost equal to the cardiac output.

611. (b). In bronchitis, there is an upward shift of the curve
In fibrosis, the slope of the curve is flatter signifying increases in pressure and work of breathing. Whereas the curve is steeper in emphysema reflecting increased lung compliance. The pressure volume loop in bronchitis reflects an increased lung volume and airway resistance shifting the curve upward.

612. (c). It is primarily used in surgical repair of aorta
DHCA or deep hypothermic circulatory arrest involves cooling of the body to temperature between 15–22°C. This is the only reliable method of neuroprotection during global ischaemia. Hypothermia increases blood viscosity 3–4 times that of normal. The cold perfusion should be continued for 20–30 minutes after the target blood temperature is reached to ensure sufficient time for cooling.

613. (d). Obesity
Various risk factors in patients undergoing CABG surgery include: Poor LV function, Advanced age, Obesity, Previous cardiac surgery, Diabetes/Renal failure

614. (a). Symptomatic heart failure with dyspnoea, fatigue and impaired exercise tolerance
- The AHA classification classifies heart failure into 4 stages
- Stage A: High-risk for heart failure: DM, HTN or coronary heart disease
- Stage B: Asymptomatic heart failure in previous MI/valvular disease
- Stage C: Symptomatic heart failure with impaired exercise tolerance and dyspnoea at rest
- Stage D: End stage heart failure refractory to medical therapy.

615. (b). 1 rem × age
The maximum allowable radiation limit in a medical worker for a lifetime is 1 rem × age or 10 mSv × age

616. (d). Reperfusion injury
Risk factors for low cardiac output syndrome (LCOS) are:
- Perioperative LV dysfunction
- Long aortic cross clamp time
- Reperfusion inury
- Inadequate cardiac surgical repair
- Valvular heart disease
- Residual cardioplegia

617. (d). Urine output <0.3 mL/kg/hr for 24 hours

	GFR criteria	Urine output
Risk	GFR decreased >25%. Creatinine increased 1.5 times	<0.5 mL/kg/hr × 6 hrs
Inury	GFR decreased >50%. Creatinine increased 2 times	<0.5 mL/kg/hr × 12 hrs
Failure	Plasma creatinine increased × 3 times	<0.3 mL/kg/hr × 24 hrs or Anuria × 12 hrs
Loss	Persistent loss of kidney function for >4 weeks	
ESRD	End stage kidney disease for >3 months	

618. (a). Increased blood pressure above the clamp
During aortic cross clamping, there is increase in blood pressure above the level of the clamp and decrease in blood pressure below the level of the clamp. Total body oxygen consumption and mixed venous oxygen saturation decrease. There is respiratory alkalosis and metabolic acidosis.

619. (c). Decreased venous return
Aortic unclamping decreases myocardial contractility and blood pressure. It causes metabolic acidosis and

decreases venous return. Cardiac output and central venous pressures are also decreased.

620. **(b). Trans-esophageal echo**

621. **(a). Abdominal obesity**

Criteria included in metabolic syndrome	
Abdominal Girth	>102 cms in men and >88 cms in women
Serum Triglycerides	> 50 mg/dL
HDL Cholesterol	<40 mg/dL in men, <50 mg/dL in women
Blood Pressure	>130/85 mm Hg
Fasting Blood Glucose	>110 mg/dL

622. **(d). Accompanied by at least 4% decrease in saturation**
Obstructive sleep apnea (OSA) is defined as reduction of airflow of atleast 50% per episode, with at least 15 such episodes per hour of sleep. Each episode should last at least for 10 seconds and be associated with at least 4% decrease in saturation.

623. **(b). Digoxin**
Digoxin is completely dependent on the kidney for its excretion. The rest are partially dependent.

624. **(d). Bile duct stricture**
Bile duct stricture, hypotension, hepatic artery ligation are some of the causes of immediate post operative jaundice. The rest are causes of delayed post operative jaundice.

625. **(c). Age >60 years**
The extended criteria for kidney donor include:
- Age >60 years
- Age 50-59 years with one of the following:
  - History of hypertension
  - Death caused by CVA
  - Pre terminal serum creatinine >1.5 mg/dL

626. **(c). Copper**

627. **(c). Core temperature >36°C**
The criteria for determination of brain death are:
- Coma, cause of death should be known
- Neuroimaging must explain the cause of coma
- No evidence of CNS depressant drugs/paralytic agents
- Absence of severe acid base, electrolyte or endocrine disturbance
- Normothermia
- Systolic BP >100 mm Hg
- No spontaneous respirations and absence of brainstem reflexes.

628. **(a). Bispectral index monitoring (BIS)**

629. **(a). Plasma volume increases 45-55%**
In pregnancy there is an increase in erythrocyte count by 20-30%. Since the increase in plasma volume exceeds the increase in erythrocytes it creates a physiological anemia of pregnancy. There is no change in central venous pressure or pulmonary capillary wedge pressure (PCWP). Platelet count is decreased by 0-10%.

630. **(c). It is also known as supine hypotension syndrome**
- Aorto-caval compression syndrome or supine hypotension syndrome is defined as a fall in MAP >15% and a reflex increase in heart rate >20 beats per minute.
- This may be accompanied by nausea, vomiting and diaphoresis.
- This syndrome is seen in pregnant women near term due to the compression of the inferior vena cava (IVC) by the gravid uterus. A reflex increase in sympathetic activity is noted resulting in increased systemic vascular resistance to maintain blood pressure within the normal range. Anesthesia worsens aortocaval compression.

631. **(b). Laparoscopic surgeries should be performed after second trimester**
Laparoscopic surgeries should be performed after second trimester Pneumoperitoneal pressures should be maintained below 12 mm Hg (<1.6 kPa) and gasless techniques should be encouraged. The end tidal and arterial CO_2 gradient should be <3 mm Hg. Minute ventilation should be maximized to avoid maternal CO_2 retention and fetal hypercarbia and acidosis. Left uterine displacement (LUD) must be maintained.

632. **(d). Rapid sequence induction should be done**
For foetal surgery, maternal FiO_2 should be >50% with an $EtCO_2$ in the range of 28-30 mm Hg. Maternal pre-oxygenation should be done for 3 minutes followed by rapid sequence induction and intubation. Left uterine displacement (LUD) must be maintained.

633. **(a). Anemia**
According to Gurd's diagnosis of fat embolism, at least one major criterion and four minor criteria are required for diagnosis.

Major	Minor
Respiratory insufficiency	Pyrexia
Petechial rash	Tachycardia
Cerebral involvement	Retinal changes
	Jaundice
	Renal changes

634. **(a). Diabetes**
Risk factors for post operative delirium are:
- Age >60 years, male sex
- Functional, physical and sensory impairment
- Polypharmacy, excess use of opioids and sedatives. Alcohol abuse
- Pain
- Poor oral intake, lack of sleep.

635. **(d). Electrolyte imbalance**
Aggressive volume replacement in the early phase of resuscitation causes a decrease in clotting factors, haematocrit and blood viscosity. Electrolyte imbalance is also seen. Too much fluid resuscitation can dilute red cell mass and decrease oxygen carrying capacity of the blood leading to hypothermia and coagulopathies.

636. **(a). Systolic blood pressure >120 mm Hg**
Goals for early resuscitation include maintaining a systolic BP of 80–100 mmHg. Other goals are to prevent increase in serum lactate and prevent the worsening of acidosis. Serum ionized calcium should be maintained in the normal range.

637. **(a). Regional anesthesia increases the risk of DVT**
Regional anesthesia decreases the risk of DVT.

638. **(c). Exploratory aparotomy surgeries**
The risk factors include:
- Reperfusion injury
- Hemorrhage with hematoma
- Casts and circular dressings
- Crush injuries

639. **(a). Keep FiO₂ at least 50%**
For prevention of an airway fire FiO$_2$ should be kept 30% or less. N$_2$O should not be used. A saline filled 50 cc syringe should be kept ready to flood the airway in case of an airway fire. Specialized endotracheal tubes meant for laser surgery should be used and the cuff should be inflated with saline or an indicator dye to alert the anesthetist in case of a cuff leak.

640. **(d). Efferent limb is via the trigeminal nerve**
Oculoardiac Reflex: Traction on extraocular muscles causes stimulation of the long and short cilary nerves through the ciliary ganglion which finally terminate in the ophthalmic division of the trigeminal nerve. This is the afferent limb. The efferent limb is via the vagus nerve which causes bradycardia. If bradycardia occurs, the surgeon should be asked to stop the surgical manipulations and atropine should be administered in 7 mic/kg increments

641. **(a). Class I lasers are safe under all conditions**
- Class I lasers are safe under all conditions
- Class II lasers are safe due to the blink reflex
- Class IIa lasers are safe up to 1000 secs of continuous viewing
- Class IIIa lasers are dangerous if viewed for longer than 2 minutes
- Class IIIb lasers can cause retinal damage with even momentary exposure
- Class IV lasers can cause ocular injury/burns.

642. **(c). Patients moving all four limbs voluntarily are given 2 points**
As per modified Aldrette score, the patient requires a minimum of 9 points to be discharged from phase 1 recovery. Total score that can be obtained is 10. Patients with a score <9 require monitoring for a few more hours in the recovery room. A patient moving all 4 limbs actively is given 2 points. A patient with BP of 20–49% of baseline is given 1 point.

643. **(c). Succinylcholine**
Intravenous succinylcholine in a dose of anything from 0.1 to 2 mg/kg will break laryngospasm. The lower dose of 0.1 mg kg^{-1} has been reported to break laryngospasm but preserve spontaneous ventilation.

644. **(a). Decreased red cell mass**
SvO$_2$ depends on O$_2$ flux = oxygen delivery (DO$_2$) - oxygen consumption (VO$_2$) O$_2$ flux = (cardiac output × (Haemoglobin concentration × SpO$_2$ × 1.34) + (PaO$_2$ × 0.003)) - VO$_2$. Normal oxygen extraction is 25–30% corresponding to a ScvO$_2$ >65%,< 65% = Impaired tissue oxygenation and >80% = High PaO$_2$; or suspect: — Cytotoxic dysoxia (e.g. cyanide poisoning, mitochrondial disease, severe sepsis) — Microcirculatory shunting (e.g. severe sepsis, liver failure, hyperthyroidism) — Left to right shunts. A low SvO$_2$ is either be due to low cardiac output, hemoglobin or low oxygen saturation.

645. **(b). Decreased functional residual capacity**
In obese people, the presence of adipose tissue around the rib cage and abdomen and in the visceral cavity loads the chest wall and reduces functional residual capacity (FRC). This recuction in FRC lead to lower oxygen reserve during pre oxygenation and early desaturation during interuption of ventilation.

646. **(b). Left recurrent laryngeal**

647. **(c). Protein low fluid in alveolar space**
ARDS can be caused by numerous conditions including sepsis, pneumonia, smoke inhalation, trauma, acute pancreatitis, eclampsia and fat embolism. It leads to a non-cardiogenic pulmonary edema where there is leak-

age of protein rich fluid into the alveoli which leads to respiratory failure. There is an acute onset and there is bilateral diffuse infiltrates on chest X-ray. There should be no evidence of cardiac failure. The hypoxia is normally refractory and high levels of oxygen are required.

648. (a). **A 35-year-old immunosuppressed female with lung infiltrates and respiratory failure**
In the properly selected patient, noninvasive positive pressure ventilation (NPPV) can have a very positive impact on outcome. For instance, it can reduce mortality in acute COPD exacerbations by one third. Delivered through a mask or nasal appliance, it can help with both oxygenation and ventilation. Contraindications include patients with altered mental status, recent esophageal anastomosis, trauma, high-aspiration risks, or those with anticipated long-term need of PPV.

649. (a). **Malignant pleural effusion**

650. (d). **Check valve**
Check valves permit only unidirectional flow of gases. These valves prevent retrograde flow of gases from the anesthesia machine or the transfer of gas from a compressed-gas cylinder at high pressure into a container at a lower pressure. Thus, these unidirectional valves will allow an empty compressed-gas cylinder to be exchanged for a full one during operation of the anesthesia machine with minimal loss of gas. The adjustable pressure- limiting valve is a synonym for a pop-off valve. A fail-safe valve is a synonym for a pressure-sensor shut off valve. The purpose of a fail-safe valve is to discontinue the flow of N_2O if the O_2 pressure within the anesthesia machine falls below 25 psi.

651. (c). **FEF 25–75%**
Pulmonary function tests are divided into tests that assess ventilatory capacity and those that assess pulmonary gas exchange. The test to assess ventilatory capacity is the FEV1/FVC ratio, maximum mid-expiratory flow (FEF 25–75%), MVV, and flow-volume curves. The most significant disadvantage of these tests is that they are dependent on patient effort. However, because the FEF 25–75% is obtained from the mid-expiratory portion of the flow-volume loop, it is least dependent on patient effort.

652. (d) **Aspartate amino transferase and Alanine amino transferase**
Serologic liver tests are broadly divided into those that evaluate liver function (prothrombin time, bilirubin, albumin), those that evaluate integrity of hepatocytes (aspartate aminotransferase or AST, alanine aminotransferase or ALT) and those that assess abnormalities of bile ducts and bile flow (bilirubin, alkaline phosphatase, gamma glutamyl transpeptidase or). Patterns of abnormal liver tests include hepatocellular (AST and ALT elevation), cholestatic (bilirubin, AP, GGT) and mixed elevations.

653. (c). **Fat Embolism**
Fat embolism (FE) is defined by the presence of fat globules in the pulmonary microcirculation regardless of clinical significance. FES describes a characteristic pattern of clinical findings that follow an insult associated with the release of fat into the circulation.
FES is most commonly associated with orthopedic trauma, with highest incidence in closed, long bone fractures of the lower extremities, particularly the femur.
Sometime after the fracture, patients develop hypoxemia and hypotension followed by confusion and a petechial rash. Chest X-ray may show new diffuse bilateral patchy infiltrates. A transthoracic echocardiogram may show right ventricular dilation and free wall hypokinesis with preserved contractility of the right ventricular apex.

654. (c). **8**

Component tested	Score
Eye response	
Eyes open spontaneously	4
Eye opening to verbal command	3
Eye opening to pain	2
No eye opening	1
Motor response	
Obeys command	6
Localises pain	5
Withdraws from pain	4
Flexion response to pain	3
Extension response to pain	2
No motor response	1
Verbal response	
Oriented	5
Confused	4
Inappropriate words	3
Incomprehensible sounds	2
No verbal response	1

655. (d). **Wake the patient up**

As per AIDAA guidelines,

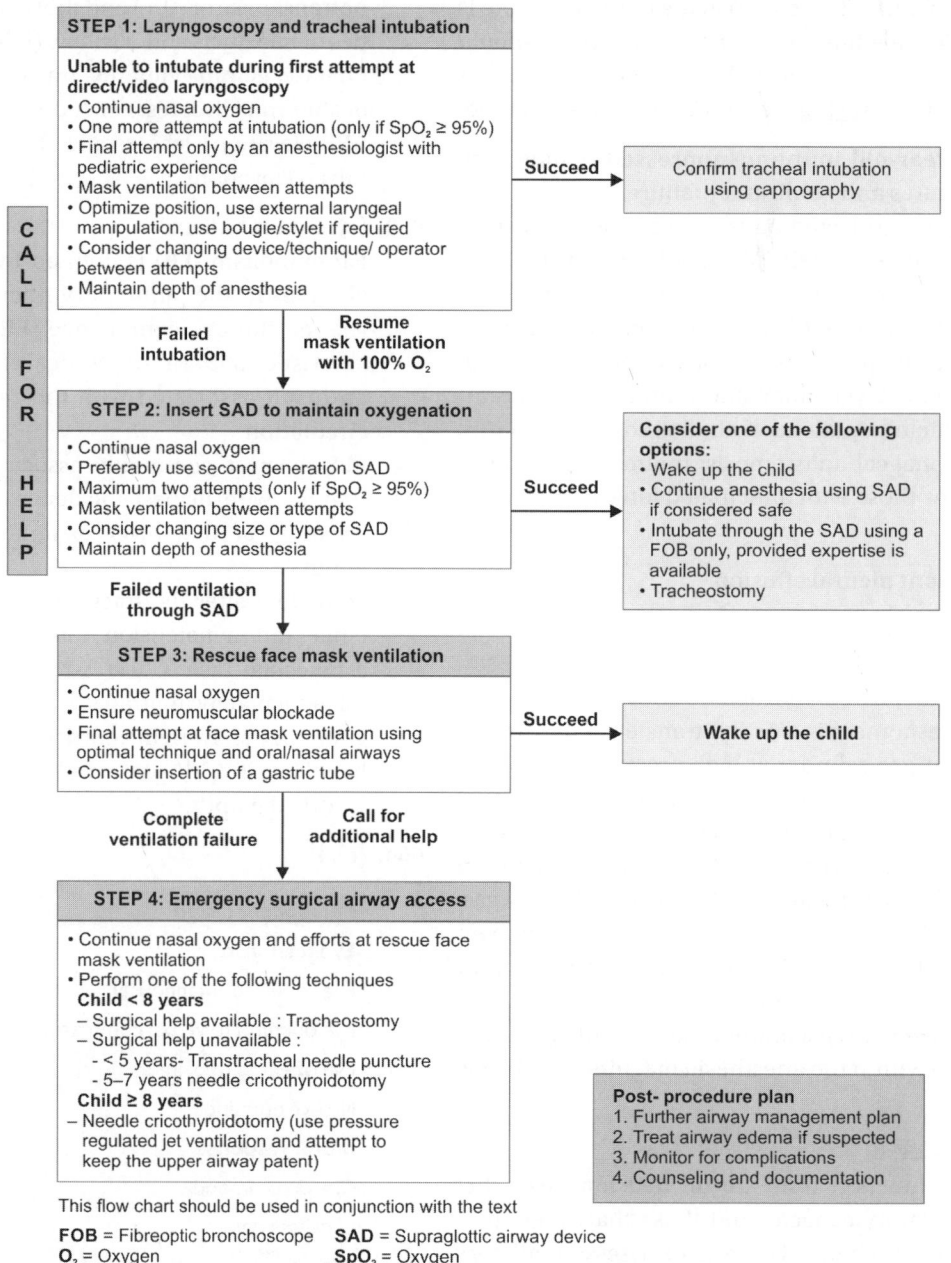

656. (b). Eliminated by plasma cholinesterase

Mivacurium is a potent nondepolarising neuromuscular blocking agent which is structurally related to the benzylisoquinolinium compound, atracurium. Mivacurium has a short duration of action due to its rapid elimination by plasma cholinesterase.

657. (c). Thiopentone

Barbiturates are mainly metabolized by the liver into inactive, water-soluble compounds by oxidation and then are renally excreted or conjugated to glucuronic acid and excreted in bile. The most significant aspect of the metabolism of barbiturates (e.g., phenobarbital, thiopental, methohexital) is their effect on the hepatic microsomal enzyme system (cytochrome P450 (CYP) enzymes). Barbiturates induce enzymes, notably δ-aminolevulinic acid (ALA) synthetase. ALA synthetase is involved in the porphyrin production pathway, and therefore barbiturates are contraindicated in patients with acute intermittent porphyria (AIP) or variegate porphyria because they may precipitate an attack, manifested by severe abdominal pain, nausea, vomiting, psychiatric disorders, and neurologic abnormalities.

658. **(b). Cocaine**
Cocaine, a powerful vasoconstrictor, induces immune responses including cytokine elevations.

659. **(d). Rectus sheath block and subcostal Transversus Abdominis Plane block**
Transversus abdominis plane block (TAP) is preferred in abdominal anterolateral wall surgeries. The TAP block is administered between the internal oblique muscle and the transverse abdominal muscle. It provides adequate analgesia in the anterior abdominal wall through the ventral branches of the nerve roots, which is divided into the ventral and dorsal rami after originating from the medulla spinalis. Compared to the TAP implemented between the costal margin and iliac crest in the sidewall of the abdomen, the analgesic effect can be increased in the interventions at upper levels like cholecystectomy with the subcostal TAP (ScTAP), which is performed at the junction of the costal arch and midclavicular line. This technique provides adequate analgesia in the middle wall of the abdomen through the block of the terminal branch of the ventral ramus.

660. **(c). Electricity**
Electricity is the driving force for the piston and so there is no requirement of a driver gas to deliver ventilation.

661. **(c). Administering inhalational agent sevoflurane and spontaneous ventilation**
Plan A should be to preserve spontaneous ventilation either by induction using IV sedative medication: propofol infusion or boluses (also dexmedetomidine, ketamine) or with Inhalation induction with Sevoflurane. While patient is spontaneously breathing, a careful insertion of the laryngoscope blade may be attempted provided that the patient tolerates without bucking nor coughing.

662. **(a). Decreased motor end-plate sensitivity to acetylcholine**
Magnesium sulfate has a pre-synaptic effect by inhibiting acetylcholine release at motor nerve terminals.

663. **(b). 71%**

664. **(c). Diplopia**
PDPH occurs with low cerebrospinal fluid volume from a leak at the site of the dural puncture that exceeds spinal fluid production resulting in low CSF pressure (intracranial hypotension). Traction precipitates symptoms on pain-sensitive structures such as the meninges, blood vessels (especially veins and sagittal or transverse sinuses), cranial nerves, and upper cervical nerves. Symptoms of PDPH include bilateral frontal or an occipital headache worse in the upright position, improved supine, associated with nausea, dizziness, neck pain, visual changes and occasionally tinnitus, hearing loss or radicular symptoms into the arms. Physical examination is usually unremarkable, and the typical patient should not exhibit fever, meningismus, altered mentation or focal neurologic findings. In unusual cases, focal findings might include nystagmus, horizontal diplopia, facial numbness or palsy.

665. **(c). Child comes to the operating room already asleep undergoing anesthesia induction without being awakened**
Steal induction is a type of inhalational induction where the child comes to the operating room already asleep undergoing anesthesia induction without being awakened. No force or physical restraint is used and the child transgresses from natural to anesthesia-induced sleep. The principle of steal induction was first described by Meyers in 1977 which used intramuscular droperidol to induce sleep. Subsequently, a number of agents have been used, including ketamine, clonidine and, more recently, melatonin.

666. **(a). Propylthiouracil**
Propylthiouracil is the preferred drug for treatment of hyperthyroidism in pregnant women because it does not cross the placenta.

667. **(d). Sciatic nerve injury**
Injury to the sciatic nerve is an infrequent but important complication of gynecologic procedures in which the lithotomy position is used.
Peroneal nerve injury will cause foot drop.

668. **(d). Infants have higher minute ventilation-to-FRC ratio**
Infants have higher alveolar ventilation and lower FRC compared to adults. This higher minute ventilation-to-FRC ratio along with higher blood flow to vessel rich organs leads to rapid rise in alveolar concentration, speeding induction.

669. **(c). Morphine**
After a drug is deposited in the epidural space, but before it reaches the spinal cord, it must first cross a hydrophilic zone (extracellular and intracellular fluids) and then a hydrophobic zone (cell membrane lipids) of the arachnoid membrane. Thus, before there is diffusion through these two areas, the drug must first dissolve in those environments. Lipophilic drugs readily dissolve in the lipophilic component of arachnoid mater and thus cross the region easily. Conversely, they penetrate the hydrophilic zone with difficulty, creating the rate-limiting factor in their diffusion through the arachnoid membrane. Drugs with intermediate lipophilicity move more readily between the lipid and the aqueous zones,

and their meningeal permeability coefficients are correspondingly greater (e.g., alfentanil, hydromorphone, meperidine). These physical and chemical properties of the opioids will also determine vascular permeability. Opioids with high octanol:buffer sufentanil, move more easily to the intravascular compartment than to the subarachnoid compartment. Thus, spinal cord concentrations of an opioid after epidural administration are the result of the net difference between the rate of uptake and distribution to the vascular and subarachnoid spaces. These differences explain why morphine, despite having a meningeal permeability coefficient similar to fentanyl and sufentanil, which are well below the optimal range of meningeal penetration, is a useful drug for epidural analgesia.

670. **(c). Decrease succinylcholine-induced fasciculations**
Magnesium sulphate can prevent and reduce the degree of fasciculations caused by succinylcholine during induction anesthesia.

671. **(b). 4 hours**
Time Remaining (hours) = Pressure (Psig)/200 × Flow rate (L/min)
Time remaining for one cylinder = 1100/(200 × 5)
= 1.1 hours
Time required for 4 cylinders = 4 × 1.1
= 4.4 hours
~ 4 hours

672. **(b). Is associated with less/almost nil histamine release**
At the same dose (2 × ED_{95} dose) atracurium is more effective neuromuscular blocking agent than cisatracurium, while higher doses of cisatracurium 4 × ED_{95} and 6 × ED_{95} provide more effective, more rapid neuromuscular blocking with longer duration of action, stable hemodynamic status, and no associated signs of histamine release clinically.

673. **(d). Isoflurane**
Isoflurane increased cerebral blood flow and decreased cerebral metabolic rate of oxygen. Desflurane reduced mean cerebral metabolic rate of oxygen ($CMRO_2$) and mean cerebral metabolic rate of glucose (CMRglc). Concomitantly, Cerebral Blood Flow was significantly reduced. Etomidate and Fentanyl both decrease Cerebral blood flow and cerebral metabolic rate.

674. **(c). Cl^-**
Strong ions are cations and anions that exist as charged particles dissociated from their partner ions at physiologic pH. Thus, these ions are "strong" because their ionization state is independent of pH.
The Strong Ion Difference (SID) is the difference between the positively- and negatively-charged strong ions and it is used to determine acid-base status of patients using the Physiochemical approach described by Stewart. Many authorities claim this approach to be better than the usual approach using the Henderson-Hasselbalch equation.

675. **(b). GP Ib-IX**
- GP VI is the receptor for collagen
- GP Ib-IX binds vWF
- GP IIb-IIIa binds fibrinogen
- GP Ia-IIa binds collagen.

676. **(a). Parecoxib**
Parecoxib is a prodrug of Valdecoxib.

677. **(d). Codeine**
Cytochrome P450 CYP2D6 is the most extensively characterized polymorphic drug-metabolizing enzyme. There are many drugs whose metabolism is catalyzed by CYP2D6. These include β-blockers (metaprolol, propranolol) Antidepressants (amitryptiline, fluoxetine), Antiarrhythmic drugs (eacainide, flecainide), neuroleptics (haloperidol, thioridazine) and Codeine, among others.

678. **(c). 0.64 and 0.77**
Damping is the process of the system absorbing the energy of oscillations. While some damping is required in all systems, excessive damping (overdamping) or insufficient damping (underdamping) will affect the output adversely.
Critical damping is the minimum amount of damping to prevent any overshoot. If a brief burst of energy is applied to a critically damped system, for example by quickly flushing an arterial line system, after displacement, the wave returns to baseline, without any overshoot. This system is relatively slow to respond.
The optimal damping coefficient will be around 0.7, which provides the best balance between speed of response and accuracy.

679. **(c). Has high hepatic extraction ratio**
A. Ketamine is a non-competitive antagonist at the NMDA receptor and binds to the phencyclidine binding site on the receptor
B. S (+) isomer produces more intense analgesia, rapid recovery, less salivation and lower incidence of emergence reactions
C. Correct. High HER, therefore clearance affected by changes in hepatic blood flow
D. Ketamine has low protein binding.

680. **(d). Palonosetron**
Palonosetron is a second generation serotonin receptor antagonist.
It has an extended half-life (approx. 40 hours), superior efficacy, does not appear to affect the QT interval and

therefore may be safer for patients at risk for cardiac arrhythmias

681. **(a). Domperidone**
Domperidone has action only on peripheral D2 receptors. Therefore, neuropsychiatric and extrapyramidal side effects are rare as compared to Metoclopramide.

682. **(b). Cytotoxic hypoxia**
The mechanism for propofol induced metabolic acidosis may reflect poisoning (cytotoxic hypoxia) of the electron transport chain and impaired oxidation of long chain fatty acids by propofol.
Lactic acidosis has been described in pediatric and adult patients receiving prolonged high dose infusions of propofol (>75 mic/kg/min) for longer than 24 hours.

683. **(b). Progesterone**
Progesterone and estrogen decrease lower esophageal tone and make reflux more likely
Anti-cholinesterases (Neostigmine) and D2 receptor antagonists (Metoclopramide and Domperidone) increase lower esophageal tone and make reflux less likely.

684. **(a). Secretin**
- Secretin delays gastric emptying
- Neostigmine and Gastrin increase gastric emptying
- Chyme with low pH delays gastric emptying

685. **(c). 1%**
A small change in osmolality (as low as 1%), can produce a large change in serum ADH concentration, thus producing a tight regulation of serum osmolality.

686. **(b). Bradycardia**
The Bezold–Jarisch reflex is a circulatory response whereby a decrease in left ventricular volume activates receptors that case a paradoxical bradycardia. This compensatory decrease in HR allows for increased ventricular filling but may also exacerbate hypotension. The bradycardia and hypotension that can occur during spinal or epidural anesthesia have been attributed to this reflex.

687. **(b). Septic shock**
Pyruvate dehydrogenase (PDH) is a key enzyme in aerobic metabolism. PDH converts pyruvate, the end product of glycolysis, into acetyl-coenzyme A, which then enters the Krebs cycle. Excess pyruvate, due to inadequate PDH, PDH inhibition, or other causes, can alternatively be converted to lactate via anaerobic metabolism. (*Mayo Clin Proc.* 2013;88:1127–1140) Sepsis causes a reduction in the activity and quantity of PDH, which has, in turn, been associated with increased levels of lactate. (*Am J Physiol.* 1991;260:E669–E674, *Shock.* 1996;6:89–94)

688. **(a). Angiotensin II**
Angiotensinogen has 485 amino acids, including a 33 amino-acid signal peptide and it is the only precursor for all angiotensins. It is converted to Angiotensin-I (a decapeptide hormone) that can be cleaved to (octapeptide) angiotensin-II. Angiotensin III is a heptapeptide formed from ANGIOTENSIN II. Angiotensin III has the same efficacy as Angiotensin in promoting Aldosterone secretion and modifying renal blood flow, but less vasopressor activity.

689. **(d). Net loss of 4 ATPs**
The Cori cycle involves the conversion of lactate to glucose in the liver, release of glucose into the blood, uptake of glucose by peripheral tissues, conversion of glucose to lactate by glycolysis, the release of lactate into the blood, and uptake of lactate by the liver for neoglucogenesis. Six ATPs are consumed in the process to deliver 2 ATPs to the peripheral tissues.

690. **(c). Increased cardiac responsiveness to catecholamines**
The effect of metabolic acidosis on the cardiovascular system varies with pH, so that at pH > 7.2 heart rate and contractility increase, but at as the pH decreases to <7.1, the contractility decreases. It also lowers the threshold for various arrhythmias. Metabolic acidosis also reduces cardiac responsiveness to various vasopressors

691. **(a). Temporal separation of injection of induction agent and muscle relaxant**
In critically ill patients who are delirious, uncooperative, and may not allow preoxygenation, the dissociate induction agent Ketamine can be given first, patient preoxygenated using bag and mask or 100% oxygen and once adequate preoxygenation is achieved, a muscle relaxant is administered and patient intubated.

692. **(d). Left ventricular failure**
The physiologically difficult airway, where the presence of physiologic derangements makes the patient vulnerable to cardiovascular collapse during airway management. The four physiologically difficult airways include hypoxemia, hypotension, severe metabolic acidosis, and right ventricular failure

693. **(d). Capnography**
While other methods may be used for confirmation of tracheal placement of the endotracheal tube, waveform capnography remains the Gold Standard for this, since all other methods have their own limitations.

694. **(d). Cormack Lehane Grade IIb view**
In the modified version of the Cormack and Lehane scoring system, while grades I, III and IV remain the

same, grade 2 (only part of the glottis visible) is divided into 2a (part of the cords visible) and 2b (only the arytenoids or the very posterior origin of the cords visible).

695. **(b). The time taken for blood plasma concentration of a drug to decline by 50% after the infusion has been stopped**

696. **(d). Concentration of phenytoin decreases in a predictable manner**
The basic difference between zero and first-order kinetics is the elimination rate as compared to total plasma concentration. Drugs with zero-order kinetics undergo constant elimination regardless of the plasma concentration and phenytoin is a prime example this, as a result the concentration of phenytoin decreases in a predictable manner. Elimination of drugs with first-order kinetics proportionally increases as the plasma concentration increases, following an exponential elimination phase as the system never achieves saturation.

697. **(c). Class III**
The American College of Surgeons Advanced Trauma Life Support (ATLS) hemorrhagic shock classification uses the correlation between the amount of blood lost to expected physiologic responses of the patient. For this Heart and respiratory rates, blood pressure, mental changes, and urine output are taken into account. In the given example the patient has Class III shock since there is an increased heart, a significant decrease in blood pressure, he is confused and the urine output is low.

698. **(d). Digoxin overdose**
Drugs and toxins which are sodium channel antagonists are cardiotoxic agents. Sodium bicarbonate is useful in the treatment of poisoning due to with sodium channel blocking agents such as Tricyclic antidepressants, cocaine, quinine, quinidine, etc. Sodium bicarbonate is also used as adjunctive therapy in poisonings due to methanol, ethylene glycol, and salicylates. Digoxin increases intracellular calcium in myocardial cells indirectly, by inhibiting the sodium–potassium pump in the cell membrane and has no effect on sodium channels. Severe digoxin toxicity is treated with digoxin-specific antibody fragments, which form complexes with the digoxin molecules, which are later excreted in urine. Sodium bicarbonate has no role in management of digoxin toxicity.

699. **(a). Uses same transducer crystals to transmit and receive ultrasound**
Systemic blood pressure can not be measured. Doppler measures pressure difference across chambers by flow measurements. E.g., Flow velocity of tricuspid regurgitation can be used to estimate. Right ventricular systolic pressure, and hence pulmonary artery pressure.
Slightest movements of probe can cause large change in measurements.
Red indicates blood flow towards and blue indicates flow away from the transducer.

700. **(c). *Enterobacter aerogenes***
Enterobacter aerogenes is gram negative.